Laboratory Manual for Strength and Conditioning

The *Laboratory Manual for Strength and Conditioning* is a comprehensive text that provides students with meaningful lab experiences in the area of strength and conditioning and applied sport science. While each lab may be conducted in a sophisticated laboratory, there are opportunities to conduct the labs in a gym or field environment without costly equipment. It is a useful resource as students prepare for a career as a strength and conditioning coach, athletic trainer, physical therapist, or personal trainer.

The *Laboratory Manual for Strength and Conditioning* is designed to be a practical guide for training students and professionals in the skills to be applied to strength and conditioning. The labs cover seven major aspects of strength and conditioning including speed, power, flexibility, agility, and fitness. The labs are practical and easy to follow with sample calculations, data tables, and worksheets to complete. Each includes suggested tasks/activities to apply the theory to real-world applications.

Students will explore assessments of strength, aerobic capacity, power output, speed, change of direction, and muscular endurance, and gain understanding in the following areas:

- Definitions of commonly used terms within the area of exploration, as well as commonly misused terms
- Assessing performance (i.e., power, strength, speed, etc.)
- Understanding laboratory- and field-based techniques for specific athlete populations
- Describing optimal methods for testing in all aspects of physical performance
- Evaluation of test results based upon sport and/or athlete normative data

The lab manual is a valuable resource for strength coaches, personal trainers, kinesiology students, and educators at the undergraduate and beginning graduate-level programs and can be used in a graduate strength and conditioning course.

Joshua Miller, DHSc, CSCS, ACSM-EP, is a Clinical Associate Professor and Director of Undergraduate Studies in the Department of Kinesiology and Nutrition at the University of Illinois Chicago.

Paul Comfort, PhD, ASCC, CSCS*D, is a Professor of Strength and Conditioning and programme leader for the MSc Strength and Conditioning at the University of Salford, UK and an adjunct professor at Edith Cowan University, Western Australia.

John McMahon, CSCS*D, ASCC, is a Reader (Associate Professor) in Sport and Exercise Biomechanics at the University of Salford, UK.

Laboratory Manual for Strength and Conditioning

Joshua Miller, Paul Comfort, and John McMahon

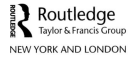

Routledge
Taylor & Francis Group

NEW YORK AND LONDON

Designed cover image: Dmytro Aksonov / Getty Images

First published 2023
by Routledge
605 Third Avenue, New York, NY 10158

and by Routledge
4 Park Square, Milton Park, Abingdon, Oxon, OX14 4RN

Routledge is an imprint of the Taylor & Francis Group, an informa business

© 2023 Joshua Miller, Paul Comfort, and John McMahon

ISBN: 978-1-032-03328-0 (hbk)
ISBN: 978-1-032-03325-9 (pbk)
ISBN: 978-1-003-18676-2 (ebk)

DOI: 10.4324/9781003186762

Typeset in Sabon LT Std
by KnowledgeWorks Global Ltd.

Contents

Figures

Tables

1 Pre-Participation Health Screening, Medical Clearance, and Informed Consent

Joshua Miller

Part 1: Introduction

Pre-participation screening is necessary to be performed prior to conducting any type of exercise training or testing because it is essential to determine if there are any medical contraindications to exercise, with risk factors, and special needs. The American College of Sports Medicine (ACSM) (ACSM, 2020) and the National Strength and Conditioning Association (NSCA) (Evetovich and Hinnerichs, 2012) recommend that all individuals complete a pre-participation screening. The goal of the screen is multifactorial: (1) to determine whether an individual has any medical condition that contraindicates performing certain fitness-related assessments, (2) to determine if an individual should have a medical evaluation before undergoing a fitness assessment and consult a physician, and (3) to determine if the participant has other health or medical concerns (i.e., orthopaedic limitations, diabetes, etc.).

The three components of the pre-participation screening include: (a) an informed consent, (b) an exercise pre-participation health screening, and (c) a medical health history (Gibson et al., 2019). This information will be used to determine if medical clearance should be obtained prior to performing any screening tests or exercise training. These documents are essential to determine the individual's current health status and the possible need for medical clearance by a physician or therapist and making sure the individual understands what will be asked of them during their participation in the exercise testing.

Informed Consent for Exercise Testing

The informed consent should be obtained first when working with a new participant (Liguori, 2018). Obtaining informed consent from a participant is an important ethical and legal consideration and should be completed prior to any collection of any personal and confidential information, any fitness testing, or exercise training. Each informed consent document may be different from one another based upon the type of testing that will be completed, the information that must be present in the informed consent should make sure that the participant understands the purpose and risks associated with screening, testing, and exercise programming. The consent form should be verbally explained, and the participant should be given the opportunity to ask as many questions they have and to be answered completely as possible prior to signing the document. It is important to document any questions the participant may have as well as the answers given. The consent should state that the participant is free to withdraw their consent at any time. In addition, all necessary steps will be taken for confidentiality of the participant. A sample informed consent is provided in Figure 1.1. It is

DOI: 10.4324/9781003186762-1

INFORMED CONSENT FOR EXERCISE TESTING

Purpose and Explanation of the Test

To assess cardiorespiratory fitness, body composition, muscular strength and endurance and flexibility, you hereby voluntarily consent to engage in one or more of the following tests (check the appropriate boxes):

◊   Body Composition Tests
◊   Graded Exercise Stress Test
◊   Muscular Strength Tests
◊   Muscular Endurance Tests
◊   Flexibility Tests

Explanation of Tests

The body composition procedure involves you sitting in an air-tight chamber while breathing normal and wearing the proper attire. You will be in the for approximately 45-seconds and then it will be repeated up to two times, if needed. This test provides an accurate estimation of your percentage body fat.

The cardiopulmonary exercise test is performed on a cycle ergometer or a treadmill. The workload is increased every few minutes until exhaustion or until other symptoms dictate that the test is terminated. You may stop the test at any time because of fatigue or discomfort. This test provides an accurate measurement of your fitness.

For muscular strength and endurance testing, you will be asked to lift weights for several repetitions using either a barbell or exercise machine. These tests will assess your muscular strength and endurance of specific muscular groups depending upon the exercise you are performing.

Your flexibility will be assessed using a Sit-and-reach box. During this test we will measure the range of motion of your lower body.

Risks and Discomforts

During the graded exercise test, we will be observing your heart rate, blood pressure, and other responses to the exercise. It has been found that irregularities can occur during exercise, and we will make every effort to minimize these situations if they occur. Emergency equipment and trained personnel are available to deal with these situations if they occur.

You may experience some claustrophobia during the Bod Pod test. However, this discomfort is momentary, but if you are unable to continue there is a button inside the device that will unlock the door immediately or you can tell the tester. If this test causes too much discomfort there are other options that we can use to estimate your body composition (e.g., skinfolds, or bioelectrical impedance).

Figure 1.1 Example of an informed consent document. *(Continued)*

There is a small possibility that you could pull a muscle or sprain a ligament during the muscular fitness (strength and endurance) testing. In addition, you could feel muscle soreness 24 or 48 hours after testing. These risks can be minimized by performing a proper warm-up prior to testing. If muscle soreness occurs, appropriate stretching exercises can aide in reducing the soreness you may feel.

Expected Benefits from Testing

These tests allow us to assess your physical fitness and to appraise you on your current physical fitness status. The results are used to prescribe a safe, sound exercise program for you. All records are kept confidential unless you consent to release this information.

Questions

Questions about the different types used in this testing battery are encouraged. If you have any questions or need additional information, please ask us to explain further or can be asked at any time during the testing.

Freedom of Consent

Your permission to perform these physical fitness tests is strictly voluntary. You are free to stop at any time if you desire.

I have read this form carefully, and I fully understand the testing procedures. I will perform knowing the risks and benefits associated. Knowing these risks and having the opportunity to ask questions that have been answered to my satisfaction, I consent to participate in the testing.

_____   _____
Signature of Patient   Date

_____   _____
Signature of Witness   Date

_____   _____
Signature of Supervisor   Date

Figure 1.1 (Continued)

suggested to have the informed consent reviewed by legal counsel. If the individual is an adolescent (< 18 years), a parent or guardian must sign in addition to the individual.

Most informed consent forms should include a statement about "emergency procedures." The personnel should be appropriately trained and authorized to carry out emergency procedures that use specific equipment. Written emergency procedures should be in place, and emergency drills should be practised at least once every 3 months, or more frequently when there is a change in staff (American College of Sports Medicine, 2018).

Procedures for Informed Consent

1   Begin administrating the Informed Consent by instructing the individual to read the document in its entirety.
2   Upon completion and prior to signing, review the document with the individual by verbally highlighting the benefits and risks associated with each test described for complete understanding.
3   Ask if he or she has any questions that they would like to answer for a particular test.
4   Upon answering all questions, ask them to sign the document. If they are an adolescent (< 18 years), ask he or she to do so and then ask their parents or guardians to sign below the signature.

Physical Activity Readiness Questionnaire for Everyone

The Physical Activity Readiness Questionnaire (PAR-Q+) (http://eparamedix.com/) was developed in Canada. It consists of a questionnaire that requires the participant to self-recall signs and symptoms that they may have or currently experience (Warburton et al., 2011). The PAR-Q+ is a widely recognized valid tool that is a safe pre-screening questionnaire for those individuals that will undertake low- to moderate-intensity exercise (Warburton et al., 2019). The seven questions are in a yes-or-no response format that are easy to understand and answer. Additionally, the PAR-Q+ has ten follow-up questions that are asked to follow-up on any of the "Yes" responses to the initial seven questions. If the individual answers "Yes" to any of the follow-up questions, he or she should be referred for medical clearance prior to testing. The questions should be followed up with the participant to make sure all questions are answered accurately and, if necessary, to ask any follow-up questions. A sample PAR-Q+ is provided in Figure 1.2.

The advantages to a PAR-Q+ are that this tool is cost effective, easy to administer, and sensitive to identify participants that may require physician clearance while not excluding those participants that would benefit from low-intensity activities (Warburton et al., 2011). There is a limitation to the use of the PAR-Q+ in that it only determines safety from exercise, but not risk of cardiovascular disease (Evetovich and Hinnerichs, 2012). Therefore, a medical health history questionnaire is completed in order to have a complete picture of the participant.

Procedures for PAR-Q+

1   Begin administrating the PAR-Q+ by instructing the individual to complete the first seven questions.

2021 PAR-Q+

The Physical Activity Readiness Questionnaire for Everyone

The health benefits of regular physical activity are clear; more people should engage in physical activity every day of the week. Participating in physical activity is very safe for MOST people. This questionnaire will tell you whether it is necessary for you to seek further advice from your doctor OR a qualified exercise professional before becoming more physically active.

GENERAL HEALTH QUESTIONS

Please read the 7 questions below carefully and answer each one honestly: check YES or NO.	YES	NO
1) Has your doctor ever said that you have a heart condition ☐ OR high blood pressure ☐?	☐	☐
2) Do you feel pain in your chest at rest, during your daily activities of living, OR when you do physical activity?	☐	☐
3) Do you lose balance because of dizziness OR have you lost consciousness in the last 12 months? Please answer NO if your dizziness was associated with over-breathing (including during vigorous exercise).	☐	☐
4) Have you ever been diagnosed with another chronic medical condition (other than heart disease or high blood pressure)? PLEASE LIST CONDITION(S) HERE: _____	☐	☐
5) Are you currently taking prescribed medications for a chronic medical condition? PLEASE LIST CONDITION(S) AND MEDICATIONS HERE: _____	☐	☐
6) Do you currently have (or have had within the past 12 months) a bone, joint, or soft tissue (muscle, ligament, or tendon) problem that could be made worse by becoming more physically active? Please answer NO if you had a problem in the past, but it does not limit your current ability to be physically active. PLEASE LIST CONDITION(S) HERE: _____	☐	☐
7) Has your doctor ever said that you should only do medically supervised physical activity?	☐	☐

☑ **If you answered NO to all of the questions above, you are cleared for physical activity.**
Please sign the PARTICIPANT DECLARATION. You do not need to complete Pages 2 and 3.

▶ Start becoming much more physically active – start slowly and build up gradually.

▶ Follow Global Physical Activity Guidelines for your age (https://www.who.int/publications/i/item/9789240015128).

▶ You may take part in a health and fitness appraisal.

▶ If you are over the age of 45 yr and NOT accustomed to regular vigorous to maximal effort exercise, consult a qualified exercise professional before engaging in this intensity of exercise.

▶ If you have any further questions, contact a qualified exercise professional.

PARTICIPANT DECLARATION
If you are less than the legal age required for consent or require the assent of a care provider, your parent, guardian or care provider must also sign this form.

I, the undersigned, have read, understood to my full satisfaction and completed this questionnaire. I acknowledge that this physical activity clearance is valid for a maximum of 12 months from the date it is completed and becomes invalid if my condition changes. I also acknowledge that the community/fitness center may retain a copy of this form for its records. In these instances, it will maintain the confidentiality of the same, complying with applicable law.

NAME _____ DATE _____

SIGNATURE _____ WITNESS _____

SIGNATURE OF PARENT/GUARDIAN/CARE PROVIDER _____

◉ **If you answered YES to one or more of the questions above, COMPLETE PAGES 2 AND 3.**

⚠ **Delay becoming more active if:**

✓ You have a temporary illness such as a cold or fever; it is best to wait until you feel better.

✓ You are pregnant - talk to your health care practitioner, your physician, a qualified exercise professional, and/or complete the ePARmed-X+ at www.eparmedx.com before becoming more physically active.

✓ Your health changes - answer the questions on Pages 2 and 3 of this document and/or talk to your doctor or a qualified exercise professional before continuing with any physical activity program.

Figure 1.2 The Physical Activity Readiness Questionnaire (PAR-Q+) for Everyone. (Reprinted with permission from the PAR-Q+ Collaboration (www.eparmedx.com) and the authors of the PAR-Q+ [Dr. Darren Warburton, Dr. Norman Gledhill, Dr. Veronica Jamnik, Dr. Roy Shephard, and Dr. Shannon Bredin].) *(Continued)*

2021 PAR-Q+

FOLLOW-UP QUESTIONS ABOUT YOUR MEDICAL CONDITION(S)

1.	**Do you have Arthritis, Osteoporosis, or Back Problems?**	
	If the above condition(s) is/are present, answer questions 1a-1c If **NO** ☐ go to question 2	
1a.	Do you have difficulty controlling your condition with medications or other physician-prescribed therapies? (Answer **NO** if you are not currently taking medications or other treatments)	YES☐ NO☐
1b.	Do you have joint problems causing pain, a recent fracture or fracture caused by osteoporosis or cancer, displaced vertebra (e.g., spondylolisthesis), and/or spondylolysis/pars defect (a crack in the bony ring on the back of the spinal column)?	YES☐ NO☐
1c.	Have you had steroid injections or taken steroid tablets regularly for more than 3 months?	YES☐ NO☐

2.	**Do you currently have Cancer of any kind?**	
	If the above condition(s) is/are present, answer questions 2a-2b If **NO** ☐ go to question 3	
2a.	Does your cancer diagnosis include any of the following types: lung/bronchogenic, multiple myeloma (cancer of plasma cells), head, and/or neck?	YES☐ NO☐
2b.	Are you currently receiving cancer therapy (such as chemotheraphy or radiotherapy)?	YES☐ NO☐

3.	**Do you have a Heart or Cardiovascular Condition? This includes Coronary Artery Disease, Heart Failure, Diagnosed Abnormality of Heart Rhythm**	
	If the above condition(s) is/are present, answer questions 3a-3d If **NO** ☐ go to question 4	
3a.	Do you have difficulty controlling your condition with medications or other physician-prescribed therapies? (Answer **NO** if you are not currently taking medications or other treatments)	YES☐ NO☐
3b.	Do you have an irregular heart beat that requires medical management? (e.g., atrial fibrillation, premature ventricular contraction)	YES☐ NO☐
3c.	Do you have chronic heart failure?	YES☐ NO☐
3d.	Do you have diagnosed coronary artery (cardiovascular) disease and have not participated in regular physical activity in the last 2 months?	YES☐ NO☐

4.	**Do you currently have High Blood Pressure?**	
	If the above condition(s) is/are present, answer questions 4a-4b If **NO** ☐ go to question 5	
4a.	Do you have difficulty controlling your condition with medications or other physician-prescribed therapies? (Answer **NO** if you are not currently taking medications or other treatments)	YES☐ NO☐
4b.	Do you have a resting blood pressure equal to or greater than 160/90 mmHg with or without medication? (Answer **YES** if you do not know your resting blood pressure)	YES☐ NO☐

5.	**Do you have any Metabolic Conditions? This includes Type 1 Diabetes, Type 2 Diabetes, Pre-Diabetes**	
	If the above condition(s) is/are present, answer questions 5a-5e If **NO** ☐ go to question 6	
5a.	Do you often have difficulty controlling your blood sugar levels with foods, medications, or other physician-prescribed therapies?	YES☐ NO☐
5b.	Do you often suffer from signs and symptoms of low blood sugar (hypoglycemia) following exercise and/or during activities of daily living? Signs of hypoglycemia may include shakiness, nervousness, unusual irritability, abnormal sweating, dizziness or light-headedness, mental confusion, difficulty speaking, weakness, or sleepiness.	YES☐ NO☐
5c.	Do you have any signs or symptoms of diabetes complications such as heart or vascular disease and/or complications affecting your eyes, kidneys, **OR** the sensation in your toes and feet?	YES☐ NO☐
5d.	Do you have other metabolic conditions (such as current pregnancy-related diabetes, chronic kidney disease, or liver problems)?	YES☐ NO☐
5e.	Are you planning to engage in what for you is unusually high (or vigorous) intensity exercise in the near future?	YES☐ NO☐

Figure 1.2 (Continued)

2021 PAR-Q+

6. **Do you have any Mental Health Problems or Learning Difficulties?** This includes Alzheimer's, Dementia, Depression, Anxiety Disorder, Eating Disorder, Psychotic Disorder, Intellectual Disability, Down Syndrome

If the above condition(s) is/are present, answer questions 6a-6b   If **NO** ☐ go to question 7

6a.	Do you have difficulty controlling your condition with medications or other physician-prescribed therapies? (Answer **NO** if you are not currently taking medications or other treatments)	YES☐ NO☐
6b.	Do you have Down Syndrome **AND** back problems affecting nerves or muscles?	YES☐ NO☐

7. **Do you have a Respiratory Disease?** This includes Chronic Obstructive Pulmonary Disease, Asthma, Pulmonary High Blood Pressure

If the above condition(s) is/are present, answer questions 7a-7d   If **NO** ☐ go to question 8

7a.	Do you have difficulty controlling your condition with medications or other physician-prescribed therapies? (Answer **NO** if you are not currently taking medications or other treatments)	YES☐ NO☐
7b.	Has your doctor ever said your blood oxygen level is low at rest or during exercise and/or that you require supplemental oxygen therapy?	YES☐ NO☐
7c.	If asthmatic, do you currently have symptoms of chest tightness, wheezing, laboured breathing, consistent cough (more than 2 days/week), or have you used your rescue medication more than twice in the last week?	YES☐ NO☐
7d.	Has your doctor ever said you have high blood pressure in the blood vessels of your lungs?	YES☐ NO☐

8. **Do you have a Spinal Cord Injury?** This includes Tetraplegia and Paraplegia

If the above condition(s) is/are present, answer questions 8a-8c   If **NO** ☐ go to question 9

8a.	Do you have difficulty controlling your condition with medications or other physician-prescribed therapies? (Answer **NO** if you are not currently taking medications or other treatments)	YES☐ NO☐
8b.	Do you commonly exhibit low resting blood pressure significant enough to cause dizziness, light-headedness, and/or fainting?	YES☐ NO☐
8c.	Has your physician indicated that you exhibit sudden bouts of high blood pressure (known as Autonomic Dysreflexia)?	YES☐ NO☐

9. **Have you had a Stroke?** This includes Transient Ischemic Attack (TIA) or Cerebrovascular Event

If the above condition(s) is/are present, answer questions 9a-9c   If **NO** ☐ go to question 10

9a.	Do you have difficulty controlling your condition with medications or other physician-prescribed therapies? (Answer **NO** if you are not currently taking medications or other treatments)	YES☐ NO☐
9b.	Do you have any impairment in walking or mobility?	YES☐ NO☐
9c.	Have you experienced a stroke or impairment in nerves or muscles in the past 6 months?	YES☐ NO☐

10. **Do you have any other medical condition not listed above or do you have two or more medical conditions?**

If you have other medical conditions, answer questions 10a-10c   If **NO** ☐ read the Page 4 recommendations

10a.	Have you experienced a blackout, fainted, or lost consciousness as a result of a head injury within the last 12 months **OR** have you had a diagnosed concussion within the last 12 months?	YES☐ NO☐
10b.	Do you have a medical condition that is not listed (such as epilepsy, neurological conditions, kidney problems)?	YES☐ NO☐
10c.	Do you currently live with two or more medical conditions?	YES☐ NO☐

PLEASE LIST YOUR MEDICAL CONDITION(S) AND ANY RELATED MEDICATIONS HERE: _____

GO to Page 4 for recommendations about your current medical condition(s) and sign the PARTICIPANT DECLARATION.

Figure 1.2 (Continued)

2021 PAR-Q+

✓ **If you answered NO to all of the FOLLOW-UP questions (pgs. 2-3) about your medical condition, you are ready to become more physically active - sign the PARTICIPANT DECLARATION below:**

▶ It is advised that you consult a qualified exercise professional to help you develop a safe and effective physical activity plan to meet your health needs.

▶ You are encouraged to start slowly and build up gradually - 20 to 60 minutes of low to moderate intensity exercise, 3-5 days per week including aerobic and muscle strengthening exercises.

▶ As you progress, you should aim to accumulate 150 minutes or more of moderate intensity physical activity per week.

▶ If you are over the age of 45 yr and **NOT** accustomed to regular vigorous to maximal effort exercise, consult a qualified exercise professional before engaging in this intensity of exercise.

◉ **If you answered YES to one or more of the follow-up questions** about your medical condition:

You should seek further information before becoming more physically active or engaging in a fitness appraisal. You should complete the specially designed online screening and exercise recommendations program - the **ePARmed-X+ at www.eparmedx.com** and/or visit a qualified exercise professional to work through the ePARmed-X+ and for further information.

⚠ **Delay becoming more active if:**

✓ You have a temporary illness such as a cold or fever; it is best to wait until you feel better.

✓ You are pregnant - talk to your health care practitioner, your physician, a qualified exercise professional, and/or complete the ePARmed-X+ **at www.eparmedx.com** before becoming more physically active.

✓ Your health changes - talk to your doctor or qualified exercise professional before continuing with any physical activity program.

● You are encouraged to photocopy the PAR-Q+. You must use the entire questionnaire and NO changes are permitted.
● The authors, the PAR-Q+ Collaboration, partner organizations, and their agents assume no liability for persons who undertake physical activity and/or make use of the PAR-Q+ or ePARmed-X+. If in doubt after completing the questionnaire, consult your doctor prior to physical activity.

PARTICIPANT DECLARATION

● All persons who have completed the PAR-Q+ please read and sign the declaration below.

● If you are less than the legal age required for consent or require the assent of a care provider, your parent, guardian or care provider must also sign this form.

I, the undersigned, have read, understood to my full satisfaction and completed this questionnaire. I acknowledge that this physical activity clearance is valid for a maximum of 12 months from the date it is completed and becomes invalid if my condition changes. I also acknowledge that the community/fitness center may retain a copy of this form for records. In these instances, it will maintain the confidentiality of the same, complying with applicable law.

NAME _____   DATE _____

SIGNATURE _____   WITNESS _____

SIGNATURE OF PARENT/GUARDIAN/CARE PROVIDER _____

──── **For more information, please contact** ────
www.eparmedx.com
Email: eparmedx@gmail.com

Citation for PAR-Q+
Warburton DER, Jamnik VK, Bredin SSD, and Gledhill N on behalf of the PAR-Q+ Collaboration. The Physical Activity Readiness Questionnaire for Everyone (PAR-Q+) and Electronic Physical Activity Readiness Medical Examination (ePARmed-X+). Health & Fitness Journal of Canada 4(2):3-23, 2011.

Key References
1. Jamnik VK, Warburton DER, Makarski J, McKenzie DC, Shephard RJ, Stone J, and Gledhill N. Enhancing the effectiveness of clearance for physical activity participation; background and overall process. APNM 36(S1):S3-S13, 2011.
2. Warburton DER, Gledhill N, Jamnik VK, Bredin SSD, McKenzie DC, Stone J, Charlesworth S, and Shephard RJ. Evidence-based risk assessment and recommendations for physical activity clearance; Consensus Document. APNM 36(S1):S266-s298, 2011.
3. Chisholm DM, Collis ML, Kulak LL, Davenport W, and Gruber N. Physical activity readiness. British Columbia Medical Journal. 1975;17:375-378.
4. Thomas S, Reading J, and Shephard RJ. Revision of the Physical Activity Readiness Questionnaire (PAR-Q). Canadian Journal of Sport Science 1992;17:4 338-345.

The PAR-Q+ was created using the evidence-based AGREE process (1) by the PAR-Q+ Collaboration chaired by Dr. Darren E. R. Warburton with Dr. Norman Gledhill, Dr. Veronica Jamnik, and Dr. Donald C. McKenzie (2). Production of this document has been made possible through financial contributions from the Public Health Agency of Canada and the BC Ministry of Health Services. The views expressed herein do not necessarily represent the views of the Public Health Agency of Canada or the BC Ministry of Health Services.

──── Copyright © 2021 PAR-Q+ Collaboration **4/ 4**
01-11-2020

Figure 1.2 (Continued)

2 If the participant answers "Yes" to one or more of the questions, instruct him or her to complete the additional ten follow-up questions. Upon review, instruct the individuals that they will be referred to their physicians for medical clearance.

3 If the participant answers "No" to the initial seven questions, he or she should be allowed to perform the exercise testing.

Health History Questionnaire or Medical History Questionnaire

All individuals must complete a health history questionnaire or medical history questionnaire (Figure 1.3) which includes questions that pertain to personal and family health history. The questionnaire should address the following questions:

- Personal illnesses, medications, surgeries, and hospitalizations
- Previous medical diagnoses and signs and symptoms of disease that are current or within the previous year, and
- Family history of heart disease, diabetes, stroke, and hypertension (high blood pressure)

Upon reviewing the responses, focus should be placed on any medical conditions that may require physician/medical clearance. If any of the responses indicate the need for physician clearance, make sure this is obtained prior to testing or starting any exercise training.

Procedures for the Health History Questionnaire

1 Begin administrating the Health History Questionnaire by instructing the individual to complete all the general information on the top of the questionnaire and all sections below.

2 Upon completion, review all questions and if further information is needed, ask follow-up questions and place their response in the margin of the document. If determined that the individual can completely perform the exercise testing safely, continue the pre-screening procedures.

If you determine there are risks that need to be addressed with medical clearance, tell the individual they will need to obtain medical clearance prior to testing.

Laboratory task: Is your athlete ready for exercise?

Complete all tasks of the pre-participation screening.

1 Administer the PAR-Q+, and Health History Questionnaire to someone in your class. Based on the results from the questionnaire, could the individual safely perform the following types of testing from the following list of types of tests. Place a check next to the appropriate test the individual could perform.

Body composition testing

Cardiopulmonary exercise testing

Muscular strength and endurance

Flexibility

Unable to perform, must obtain medical clearance prior to testing

Demographic Information

Last name	First name	Middle initial

Date of birth	Sex	Home phone

Address	City, State	Zip code

Work phone	Family physician

Section 1

1. When was the last time you had a physical examination?

2. If you are allergic to any medications, foods, or other substances, please name them.

3. If you have been told that you have any chronic or serious illnesses, please list them.

4. Give the following information pertaining to the last three times you have been hospitalized. *Note:* Women, donot list normal pregnancies.

	Hospitalization 1	Hospitalization 2	Hospitalization 3
Reason for hospitalization	_____	_____	_____
Month and year of hospitalization	_____	_____	_____
Hospital	_____	_____	_____
City and state	_____	_____	_____

Section B

During the past 12 months

1. Has a physician prescribed any form of medication for you? ☐Yes ☐No
2. Has your weight fluctuated more than a few pounds? ☐Yes ☐No
3. Did you attempt to bring about this weight change through diet or exercise? ☐Yes ☐No
4. Have you experienced any faintness, light-headedness, or blackouts? ☐Yes ☐No
5. Have you occasionally had trouble sleeping? ☐Yes ☐No
6. Have you experienced any blurred vision? ☐Yes ☐No
7. Have you had any severe headaches? ☐Yes ☐No
8. Have you experienced chronic morning cough? ☐Yes ☐No
9. Have you experienced any temporary change in your speech pattern, such asslurring or loss of speech? ☐Yes ☐No
10. Have you felt unusually nervous or anxious for no apparent reason? ☐Yes ☐No
11. Have you experienced unusual heartbeats such as skipped beats or palpitations? ☐Yes ☐No
12. Have you experienced periods in which your heart felt as though it were racingfor no apparent reason? ☐Yes ☐No

Figure 1.3 Example of a medical health history questionnaire. *(Continued)*

At present

1. Do you experience shortness or loss of breath while walking with others your own age?   ❑Yes ❑No

2. Do you experience sudden tingling, numbness, or loss of feeling in your arms, hands, legs, feet, or face?   ❑Yes ❑No

3. Have you ever noticed that your hands or feet sometimes feel cooler than other parts of your body?   ❑Yes ❑No

4. Do you experience swelling of your feet and ankles?   ❑Yes ❑No

5. Do you get pains or cramps in your legs?   ❑Yes ❑No

6. Do you experience any pain or discomfort in your chest?   ❑Yes ❑No

7. Do you experience any pressure or heaviness in your chest?   ❑Yes ❑No

8. Have you ever been told that your blood pressure was abnormal?   ❑Yes ❑No

9. Have you ever been told that your serum cholesterol or triglyceride level was high?   ❑Yes ❑No

10. Do you have diabetes?   ❑Yes ❑No

     If yes, how is it controlled?

     ❑Dietary means   ❑Insulin injection

     ❑Oral medication ❑Uncontrolled

11. How often would you characterize your stress level as being high?

     ❑Occasionally   ❑Frequently   ❑Constantly

12. Have you ever been told that you have any of the following illnesses?   ❑Yes ❑No

❑Myocardial infarction	❑Arteriosclerosis	❑Heart disease	❑Thyroid disease
❑Coronary thrombosis	❑Rheumatic heart	❑Heart attack	❑Heart valve disease
❑Coronary occlusion	❑Heart failure	❑Heart murmur	
❑Heart block	❑Aneurysm	❑Angina	

13. Have you ever had any of the following medical procedures?   ❑Yes ❑No

     ❑Heart surgery   ❑Pacemaker implant

     ❑Cardiac catheterization ❑Defibrillator

     ❑Coronary angioplasty ❑Heart transplantation

Section 3

Has any member of your immediate family been treated for or suspected to have had any of these conditions? Please identify their relationship to you (father, mother, sister, brother, etc.).

     A. Diabetes

     B. Heart disease

     C. Stroke

     D. High blood pressure

Figure 1.3 (Continued)

2 Administer the Informed Consent to the same individual that you completed question 1 in the activities. Properly describe and explain the tests that individual is able to perform based upon the PAR-Q+ and Health History Questionnaire.

Body composition testing

Cardiopulmonary exercise testing

Muscular strength and endurance

Flexibility

Unable to perform, must obtain medical clearance prior to testing

3 Complete the PAR-Q+ and Health History Questionnaire on yourself. Based upon the results, determine which types of tests are you able to complete or must obtain medical clearance.

References

American College of Sports Medicine. 2018. Emergency planning and policies. In: Sanders, M. E. (ed). *ACSM's Health/Fitness Facility Standards and Guidelines*. Champaign, IL: Human Kinetics.

Evetovich, T. K. & Hinnerichs, K. R. 2012. Client consultation and health appraisal. In: Coburn, J. W. & Malek, M. H. (eds). *NSCA's Essentials of Personal Training*, 2nd ed. Champaign, IL: Human Kinetics.

Gibson, A. L., Wagner, D. R. & Heyward, V. H. 2019. Physical activity, health, and chronic disease. In: *Advanced Fitness Assessment and Exercise Prescription*. Champaign, IL: Human Kinetics.

Liguori, G. 2018. *ACSM's Health-Related Physical Fitness Assessment Manual*. Baltimore, MD: Wolters Kluwer.

Warburton, D., Jamnik, V., Bredin, S., Shephard, R. & Gledhill, N. 2019. The 2020 physical activity readiness questionnaire for everyone (PAR-Q+) and electronic physical activity readiness medical examination (ePARmed-X+). *HFJC*, 12(4), 58–61.

Warburton, D. E. R., Gledhill, N., Bredin, S. S. D., Mckenzie, D. C., Charlesworth, S. & Shephard, R. J. 2011. The physical activity readiness questionnaire for everyone (PAR-Q+) and electronic physical activity readiness medical examination (ePARmed-X+): Summary of consensus panel recommendations. *HFJC*, 4, 26–37.

Warburton, D., Jamnik, V. & Bredin, S., et al. 2011. Evidence-based risk assessment and recommendations for physical activity clearance: An introduction. *Appl Physiol Nutr Metab*, 36 (Suppl 1), S1–2.

2 Athlete Needs Analysis

Paul Comfort and John McMahon

Part 1: Introduction

A needs analysis consists of two key components: the identification of the demands of the sport followed by the evaluation of the athlete(s), with the latter used to determine if their physical characteristics meet the required demands of the sport and subsequently identify short-term and long-term training goals. It is worth noting that some important points need to be considered when determining these physical characteristics, including age, sex, and level of competition. For team sports, differences in style of play and fixture schedules may also need to be considered, with further considerations for the differences in competition demands if the athlete competes domestically and for a national team where the demands notably increase. Such considerations help to ensure that the comparisons drawn are fair and appropriate so that the athlete is appropriately prepared for competition.

It is important to note that most published normative data include means and standard deviations alone, which do not reflect any extremes in performance. For example, when considering the total match distances covered in elite female soccer, Trewin et al. (2018) reported a squad average of $10,368 \pm 952$ m; however, based on these data, the maximum distance could be ~12,272 m and the minimum distance could be ~8,464 m, with this difference exceeding the smallest worthwhile change (1.8%) that has been reported for this metric. The differences in average total match distance between positions within soccer were also greater than the smallest worthwhile change, highlighting the importance of considering the position that the athlete plays. It is also recommended that, where possible, the strength and conditioning coach consider the "normal" distance, volume of high-speed running, number of sprints, etc., for the individual athlete, based on their own data.

Total distance covered and total relative distance (relative to time) covered are the two most common match variables reported for soccer (Miguel et al., 2021). It should be noted, however, that relative distance (distance/time played) is actually average speed and really should be referred to as such. While the total distance and average heart rate are important when considering the aerobic demands of the sport, the activities which make up this distance (e.g., accelerations, decelerations, changes of direction, and repeated high-intensity efforts) are also extremely important to understand when considering the overall demands of the sport and the physical characteristics of the athlete. To put this in context, average heart rate in a game of soccer is usually reported to be ~85% maximum heart rate, but when an average of 12 km is covered over a 90-minute duration, this results in an average speed of

DOI: 10.4324/9781003186762-2

$8 \text{ km} \cdot \text{hr}^{-1}$, which in well-trained athletes would not result in such high heart rates. It is the fact that there are multiple accelerations, decelerations, and changes of direction that elicit such high heart rates, and during some periods of repeated high-intensity activities, athletes will experience near-maximal heart rates.

Needs Analysis of the Sport

Initially it is important to determine the key performance indicator(s) (KPIs) for the sport. For some sports, where the performance outcome is based on time, distance, or weight lifted, the KPIs may be easier to determine. In such examples, it may be possible to develop a deterministic model to predict such outcomes, with additional consideration of how such performance outcomes are likely to change over time, based on previous national and world records. This is especially important for Olympic sports where quadrennial planning for the next Olympic Games is commonplace.

In sports where athletes are subjectively scored (e.g., figure skating, gymnastics, and surfing), determining performance outcomes becomes more difficult; however, if additional rotations in a task enhance the skill requirement/difficulty, then determining the requirements of the specific tasks is possible, which can then aid in the development of physical training priorities, as demonstrated in surfing (Secomb et al., 2015; Tran et al., 2015; Parsonage et al., 2017). For example, if a surfer can increase the height that they jump during skilled tasks, this results in additional time for increased rotations, which increases the difficulty of the task and therefore the associated score, as long as the style/technique is not compromised.

In team sports, due to the complex interaction between players, teams, environment, etc., the approach used to identify the requirements of the sport is usually based on the physical demands of the sport, which is usually based on the movement demands (usually derived via Global Positioning System [GPS], accelerometry, and time motion capture) and ideally heart rate data during competition. Such data commonly includes total distance covered, mean and peak heart rate, number of accelerations and decelerations, and changes of direction (some consideration may be given to the common angles of change of direction as this increases the demands of the task), and average sprint distance, along with distance covered at specific velocities (these can be expressed as arbitrary values or relative to the athlete's maximum speed). One should be mindful that exact data varies between certain sports, for example, field- vs. court-based sports and that the sampling frequency of accelerometers and GPS will affect the accuracy of the data especially for short-duration events (Portas et al., 2010; Scott et al., 2016; Huggins et al., 2020). In collision sports (e.g., rugby union, rugby league, and football), the number of impacts/collisions/tackles and the magnitude of these events may also be reported, as such actions affect recovery times post game and the requirement for additional body mass (Austin et al., 2011; Mclellan et al., 2011; Mclellan and Lovell, 2012; Mclellan and Lovell, 2013; Fullagar et al., 2017; Colomer et al., 2020).

Athlete Needs Analysis

A battery of assessments to reliably evaluate the athletes' physical characteristics is usually required to evaluate the athletes' physical capability in relation to the demands of the sport. Such testing batteries usually include assessment of aerobic capacity, force production characteristics, and objective assessments of sport-specific tasks, for example, in field-based sports, this may include short-sprint performance (e.g., 5-,

Table 2.1 Example assessment methods for evaluating different force production characteristics.

Force production characteristic	Maximum force production	Ballistic force production	Reactive force production
Assessment methods	1 RM Isometric mid-thigh pull Isometric squat	Squat jump CMJ Loaded CMJ Force-velocity profiles	Drop jump Single leg drop jump 10–5 jump test
Chapter location	6	7	7

1 RM = One Repetition Maximum; CMJ = Countermovement Jump.

10-, 20-, and 40-m sprint times), change of direction performance (e.g., 5-0-5 change of direction times) and jump performance (e.g., countermovement jump height). Force production characteristics can be divided into numerous categories (Table 2.1), with multi-joint isometric assessments also permitting calculation of rapid force production (e.g., force at specific time-points [100 ms, 150 ms, 200 ms, and 250 ms] and rate of force development over specific epochs [0–150 ms, 0–200 ms, and 0–250 ms]).

The selection of relevant tests is usually determined based on four key factors: (1) the assessment of the characteristics which align with the demands of the sport, (2) testing methods included in published research to provide benchmarks, (3) the reliability and validity of the methods (see Chapter 4), and (4) the facilities and equipment available (Figure 2.1). If the testing methods are not valid or reliable, or there is simply no research regarding the validity or reliability of the testing methods (and you are unable to determine the validity and reliability of the methods for yourself), it is advisable to select a different testing method. It is also important to consider the measurement error associated with the testing method and the variables of interest so that you can determine if observed changes in the future are greater than the associated measurement error, especially for individual athlete performances. Validity, reliability, and measurement error are discussed in more detail in Chapter 4.

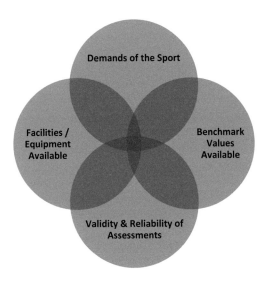

Figure 2.1 Considerations for the selection of physical performance tests.

If normative or benchmark data is available for comparisons to be made, it is important to consider if the benchmarks are for a comparable group of athletes, in terms of level of competition, age, and sex, to ensure that fair comparisons are made. It is also important to ensure that the methods of assessment and data analyses that were employed to compile any published normative data reflect those used when assessing your athletes. If using the data for longitudinal planning, then consideration for older age groups or a higher level of competition may be relevant. However, when published benchmark data is not available, it may be appropriate to set performance criteria based on the ranges observed within the squad, in relation to the demands of the sport and/or positional groups.

Data Analysis and Interpretation

Including several fitness tests as part of athlete fitness-testing batteries results in the accumulation of many different types of data, many with different units of measurement. To overcome the difficulty of presenting several fitness test results to athletes and coaches, there is a potential benefit of reporting the results in a standardised form (McMahon et al., 2021). Specifically, the calculation of standardised scores, such as the z-score, standard ten score, percentiles, or t-score will likely aide the athletes' understanding of how they have performed for a range of potentially complex fitness test results. The z-score is commonly reported by many fitness test software manufacturers. It tells us how many standard deviations an individual athlete's test score is from the mean test score (either the squad mean or a normative data mean). It is calculated using the following formula (McGuigan et al., 2013; Lockie et al., 2018):

$$\text{z-score} = \text{(the individual athlete's test score} - \text{the squad or normative data mean [average] test score)} \div \text{the squad or normative data standard deviation for the test score}$$

One assumption of the z-score calculation is that the squad or normative data mean and standard deviation values are normally distributed. Another assumption of the z-score calculation is that the sample size (i.e., number of individual athletes' data) from which the squad or normative data mean and standard deviation are derived is ≥ 30 (Turner et al., 2019). Most z-scores range between -3 and 3 by accounting for ~99.7% of normally distributed values (Turner et al., 2019). T-scores are arguably more intuitive for most non-statistically trained athletes as they avoid the use of small and often negative numbers and instead provide a score for each fitness test out of a maximum of 100 (e.g., a 0–100 scale). T-scores can be easily calculated from the z-score using the following formula:

$$T = (\text{z} - \text{score} \times 10) + 50$$

Turner et al. (2019) also highlight that t-scores, if preferred to z-scores, can be calculated directly from any fitness test score by using the following formula:

$$\text{t-score} = 50 + 10 \times ((\text{the individual athlete's test score} - \text{the squad or normative data mean [average] test score)} \div \text{the squad or normative data standard deviation for the test score)}$$

Table 2.2 A comparison of T-score, z-score, standard ten and percentile values.

Description	T-Score	Z-Score	STEN	Percentile
Excellent	>80	>3.0	>10.0	>99.9
Very Good	70	2.0	9.5	97.7
Good	60	1.0	7.5	84.1
Above Avg.	55	0.5	6.5	69.1
Average (Avg.)	50	0.0	5.5	50.0
Below Avg.	45	−0.5	4.5	30.9
Poor	40	−1.0	2.5	6.7
Very Poor	30	−2.0	0.5	0.6
Extremely Poor	<20	<−3.0	0.0	<0.1

Examples of presenting T-scores for a range of performance metrics on a radar chart with an integrated traffic light system approach have been reported in both a recent book (McMahon et al., 2022b) and peer-reviewed study McMahon et al. (2022a). Also, a framework for constructing performance bands from T-scores was recently proposed which includes suggested qualitative terms to describe the different performance bands (McMahon, 2022, McMahon and Comfort, 2022). The qualitative descriptions, ranged from extremely poor to excellent, based on the T-score range, are as follows: <20 (extremely poor), ≥20 to ≤30 (very poor), >30 to ≤40 (poor), >40 to ≤45 (below average), >45 to ≤55 (average), >55 to ≤60 (above average), >60 to ≤70 (good), >70 to ≤80 (very good), and >80 (excellent) (McMahon, 2022). This approach, shown in Table 2.2, alongside the corresponding z-score, standard ten, and percentile values, may be considered by strength and conditioning coaches who wish to standardise their athlete's test results and create benchmarks.

Part 2: Example 1 – Women's Soccer Needs Analysis

Match Demands

Elite female soccer players generally cover ~10 km in a match, although this varies depending on the position and style of play (Datson et al., 2017; Trewin et al., 2018; Randell et al., 2021). More important are the actions and activities that collectively make up the total distance covered, including high-speed running (347–2,917 m), total sprinting distance (98–850 m), maximal running speed accelerations, and decelerations (Datson et al., 2014; Randell et al., 2021), with high-intensity running and sprinting making up ~25% of the total distance covered (Vescovi and Favero, 2014), as these may be better related to successful match outcomes (Randell et al., 2021). The pattern of such high-intensity activities is also essential, as the "worst-case scenario," which constitutes the most demanding theoretical period of a match based on repeated high-intensity efforts, has not been described within the literature (Datson et al., 2019; Randell et al., 2021).

Physical Characteristics

Key physical characteristics are presented in Table 2.3. The characteristics represent some of the commonly conducted tests to evaluate important physical characteristics in elite female soccer. Remember that the mean is simply the average of the

Table 2.3 Commonly reported physical characteristics of elite female soccer players, from published data.

Physical characteristics	Range	Mean ± standard deviation
Height (m)	1.61–1.70	
Body Mass (kg)	56.6–65.1	
Body Fat (%)	14.5–22.0	
VO_{2max} (ml·kg^{-1}·min^{-1})	49.8–57.6	
Yoyo Intermittent Recovery Test, Level 1 (m)	600–1,960	1,224 ± 255
Yoyo Intermittent Endurance Test, Level 2 (m)		1,774 ± 532
Sprint 5 m (s)		1.14 ± 0.04
Time* 10 m (s)		1.91 ± 0.04
20 m (s)		3.17 ± 0.03
Countermovement Jump Height (cm)		26.1 ± 4.8 to 51.0 ± 5.0 (Commonly reported average ~35 cm)
Isometric Mid-Thigh Pull, Relative Peak Force (N·kg^{-1})#		28.5 ± 2.2

Source: Data obtained from Datson et al. (2014), Randell et al. (2021), and Emmonds et al. (2020).

Varying methodologies may have been used to collect this data across numerous studies.

* Sprint times are from research >10 years old and physical performances have improved over the last decade, although there is a lack of published data in elite female soccer players.

\# Based on youth athletes – as no data is available for senior female soccer players.

squad and that ± one standard deviation represents 68% of the athletes' data and ± two standard deviations represent 95% of the athletes' data who make up the cohort included (based on normally distributed data – see detailed discussion about this in Chapter 4). Other characteristics, such as a change of direction performance or rebound jump performance, may also be beneficial to consider when evaluating female soccer athletes' training needs.

Injury Considerations

Adult female soccer players demonstrate an incidence of 6.1 injuries per 1,000 hours of playing time, with the incidence six to seven times higher in competition compared to training. These injuries are more commonly non-contact in nature, occurring in the lower limbs, with the ankle and knee being the most common sites and muscle, tendon, and ligament injuries most prevalent (Randell et al., 2021). The fact that the majority of the injuries are non-contact highlights the potential to decrease injury risk with appropriate training interventions.

Identification of Training Priorities (Short- and Long-Term)

Table 2.4 presents the physical characteristics of a female soccer player, which you should compare to the normative data in Table 2.3, while considering the demand for the sport, to determine the athlete's training priorities. Both short-term (e.g., 4–8 weeks) and long-term (e.g., annual) goals should be identified, prioritised, and then appropriately sequenced, so that the culmination of the short-term goals should ensure attainment of the long-term goals.

Table 2.4 Athlete characteristics – case study 1.

Physical characteristic		Value/performance	Normative data	Evaluation (✓/✗)
Height (m)		1.65		
Body Mass (kg)		55.0		
Body Fat (%)		15.3		
VO$_{2max}$ (ml·kg^{-1}·min^{-1})		56.5		
Yoyo Intermittent Recovery Test, Level 1 (m)		1900		
Sprint Time	5 m (s)	1.21		
	10 m (s)	2.02		
	20 m (s)	3.25		
Countermovement Jump Height (cm)		36.5		
Isometric Mid-Thigh Pull, Peak Force (N)		1,250		

Short-Term Goals

1 –
2 –
3 –
4 –

Long-Term Goals

a)
b)
c)

Sequencing of Short-Term Goals to Achieve Long-Terms Goals

Part 3: Example 2 – Basketball Needs Analysis

Game Demands

Basketball is a physically demanding team sport in which athletes have to repeatedly accelerate, decelerate, change direction, and jump (~40 × per game) throughout the four quarters of the game (Stojanović et al., 2018; García et al., 2020). Interestingly, rapid decelerations (>3 m·s^{-2}) occur more frequently (3.2 ± 0.7 to 4.5 ± 1.4 per minute, depending on position) than rapid accelerations (0.8 ± 0.3 to 1.5 ± 0.4 per minute, depending on position), while the number of moderate accelerations (<3 m·s^{-2}) exceeds the number of moderate decelerations (Vázquez-Guerrero et al., 2018), highlighting an important consideration for training to enhance performance and mitigate injury risk. While the distances of the accelerations are generally short, athletes reach peak speeds of between 20 and 22 km·hr⁻¹ (García et al., 2020). In contrast to other team sports, such as soccer, the total distances covered are dramatically lower (5–6 km). However, this is over only a 40-minute duration, resulting in heart rates >85% maximum heart rate (Stojanović et al., 2018).

Interestingly, there is a general trend of a decrease in speed, distance covered, accelerations, and decelerations across the four quarters of a game (Stojanović et al., 2018; Vázquez-Guerrero et al., 2018; García et al., 2020; García et al., 2021), highlighting the importance of a high aerobic capacity to permit rapid recovery between the high-intensity efforts across the game. Stojanović et al. (2018) also highlight that there are differences between positional demands and that there are notable differences in game demands between countries, both of which should be considered when determining "benchmarks" and comparing to published "norms."

Physical Characteristics

Key physical characteristics are presented in Table 2.5. The characteristics represent some of the commonly conducted tests to evaluate important physical characteristics of collegiate and professional basketball. Remember that the mean is simply the average of the squad and that ± one standard deviation represents 68% of the athletes' data and ± two standard deviations represent 95% of the athletes' data who make up the cohort included (based on normally distributed data – see detailed discussion about this in Chapter 4). Other characteristics, such as change of direction performance or rebound jump performance, may also be beneficial to consider when evaluating basketball athletes' training needs. Additionally, some of these data are from rather old studies, although much of this information is the most up-to-date information available.

Injury Considerations

Between 58% and 66% of basketball injuries are sustained to the legs, consisting of non-contact and traumatic injuries (Taylor et al., 2015). These tend to be predominantly ankle and knee ligament injuries; however, anterior cruciate ligament injuries

Table 2.5 Commonly reported physical characteristics of collegiate and professional basketball players, from published data.

Physical characteristics	Range	Mean ± standard deviation
Height (m)	1.75–2.28	
Body Mass (kg)	64.0–116.0	
Body Fat (%)	5.5–20.1	
VO_{2max} (ml·kg⁻¹·min⁻¹)	50–60	
40-yard Sprint Time		4.81 ± 0.26
Countermovement Jump Height (cm)	36.1–83.0	Forwards – 57.8 ±6.5
		Centres – 54.6 ± 6.9
		Guards – 59.6 ± 9.6
1-RM Back Squat – Absolute (kg) and relative (kg·kg⁻¹)		Absolute – 152.2 ± 36.5
		Relative – 1.67 ± 0.47

Source: Data from Latin et al. (1994) Berg and Latin (1995) Ostojic et al. (2006) and Ziv and Lidor (2009).
Varying methodologies may have been used to collect this data across numerous studies.

Table 2.6 Athlete characteristics – case study 2.

Physical Characteristic	Value/Performance	Normative Data	Evaluation (✓/✗)
Height (m)	2.05		
Body Mass (kg)	118		
Body Fat (%)	21.2		
VO_{2max} ($ml \cdot kg^{-1} \cdot min^{-1}$)	48.5		
40-yard Sprint Time	5.01		
Countermovement Jump Height (cm)	56.5		
1 RM Back Squat (kg)	105		

are of great concern as the incidence is notably higher than in most other sports (Agel et al., 2005). The fact that the majority of the injuries are non-contact highlights the potential to decrease injury risk with appropriate training interventions focusing on strengthening and appropriate movement mechanics during deceleration during landing and change of direction tasks (Herrington, 2010; Myer et al., 2012; Taylor et al., 2015; Herrington et al., 2015).

Identification of Training Priorities (Short- and Long-Term)

Table 2.6 presents the physical characteristics of a male collegiate basketball player, which you should compare to the normative data in Table 2.5, while considering the demands of the sport, to determine the athlete's training priorities. Both short-term (e.g., 4–8 weeks) and long-term (e.g., annual) goals should be identified, prioritised, and then appropriately sequenced so that the culmination of the short-term goals should ensure attainment of the long-term goals.

Short-Term Goals

1 –
2 –
3 –
4 –

Long-Term Goals

a)
b)
c)

Sequencing of Short-Term Goals to Achieve Long-Terms Goals

References

Agel, J., Arendt, E. A. & Bershadsky, B. 2005. Anterior cruciate ligament injury in national collegiate athletic association basketball and soccer: A 13-year review. *Am J Sports Med*, 33, 524–30.

Austin, D. J., Gabbett, T. J. & Jenkins, D. J. 2011. Repeated high-intensity exercise in a professional rugby league. *J Strength Cond Res*, 25, 1898–904.

Berg, K. & Latin, R. W. 1995. Comparison of physical and performance characteristics of NCAA division I basketball and football players. *J Strength Cond Res*, 9(1), 22–6.

Colomer, C. M. E., Pyne, D. B., Mooney, M., Mckune, A. & Serpell, B. G. 2020. Performance analysis in rugby union: A critical systematic review. *Sports Med Open*, 6, 4.

Datson, N., Drust, B., Weston, M. & Gregson, W. 2019. Repeated high-speed running in elite female soccer players during international competition. *Sci Med Footb*, 3, 150–6.

Datson, N., Drust, B., Weston, M., Jarman, I. H., Lisboa, P. J. & Gregson, W. 2017. Match physical performance of elite female soccer players during international competition. *J Strength Cond Res*, 31, 2379–87.

Datson, N., Hulton, A., Andersson, H., Lewis, T., Weston, M., Drust, B. & Gregson, W. 2014. Applied physiology of female soccer: An update. *Sports Med*, 44, 1225–40.

Emmonds, S., Sawczuk, T., Scantlebury, S., Till, K. & Jones, B. 2020. Seasonal changes in the physical performance of elite youth female soccer players. *J Strength Cond Res*, 34.

Fullagar, H. H. K., Mccunn, R. & Murray, A. 2017. Updated review of the applied physiology of American College Football: Physical demands, strength and conditioning, nutrition, and injury characteristics of America's favorite game. *Int J Sports Physiol Perform*, 12, 1396–403.

García, F., Castellano, J., Reche, X. & Vázquez-Guerrero, J. 2021. Average game physical demands and the most demanding scenarios of basketball competition in various age groups. *J Hum Kinet*, 79, 165–74.

García, F., Vázquez-Guerrero, J., Castellano, J., Casals, M. & Schelling, X. 2020. Differences in physical demands between game quarters and playing positions on professional basketball players during official competition. *J Sports Sci Med*, 19, 256–63.

Herrington, L. 2010. The effects of 4 weeks of jump training on landing knee valgus and crossover hop performance in female basketball players. *J Strength Cond Res*, 24, 3427–32.

Herrington, L., Munro, A. & Comfort, P. 2015. A preliminary study into the effect of jumping-landing training and strength training on frontal plane projection angle. *Man Ther*, 20, 680–5.

Huggins, R. A., Giersch, G. E. W., Belval, L. N., Benjamin, C. L., Curtis, R. M., Sekiguchi, Y., Peltonen, J. & Casa, D. J. 2020. The validity and reliability of global positioning system units for measuring distance and velocity during linear and team sport simulated movements. *J Strength Cond Res*, 34, 3070–7.

Latin, R. W., Berg, K. & Baechle, T. 1994. Physical and performance characteristics of NCAA division I male basketball players. *J Strength Cond. Res*, 8, 214–18.

Lockie, R. G., Risso, F. G., Giuliano, D. V., Orjalo, A. J. & Jalilvand, F. 2018. Practical fitness profiling using field test data for female elite-level collegiate soccer players: A case analysis of a division I team. *Strength Cond J*, 40, 58–71.

McGuigan, M. R., Cormack, S. J. & Gill, N. D. 2013. Strength and power profiling of athletes: Selecting tests and how to use the information for program design. *Strength Cond J*, 35, 7–14.

Mclellan, C. P. & Lovell, D. I. 2012. Neuromuscular responses to impact and collision during elite rugby league match play. *J Strength Cond Res*, 26, 1431–40.

Mclellan, C. P. & Lovell, D. I. 2013. Performance analysis of professional, semi-professional and junior elite rugby league match-play using global positioning systems. *J Strength Cond Res*, 27, 3266–74.

Mclellan, C. P., Lovell, D. I. & Gass, G. C. 2011. Performance analysis of elite rugby league match play using global positioning systems. *J Strength Cond Res*, 25, 1703–10.

McMahon, J.J. Turner, A.N. & Comfort, P. 2021. Analysis and presentation of fitness test results. In: Turner, A.N. & Comfort, P. (eds) *Advanced Strength and Conditioning: An evidence Based Approach*. 2nd ed. Routledge. pp. 176–189.

Mcmahon, J. J. 2022. *Future Considerations for Contextualising Force Plate Test Results in Professional Football*, 31st August European College of Sport Science Congress. Seville, Spain.

Mcmahon, J. J. & Comfort, P. 2022. Countermovement jump take-off momentum benchmarks for professional rugby league forwards and backs. British Association of Sport and Exercise Sciences Biomechanics Interest Group Annual Meeting, 25th May, 2022, On-line.

Mcmahon, J. J., Lake, J. P. & Comfort, P. 2022a. Identifying and reporting position-specific countermovement jump outcome and phase characteristics within rugby league. *PLOS One*, 17, e0265999.

Mcmahon, J. J., Turner, A. N. & Comfort, P. 2022b. Analysis and presentation of fitness test results. In: Turner, A. N. & Comfort, P. (eds). *Advanced Strength and Conditioning: An Evidence-Based Approach*. 2 ed. London, UK: Routledge.

Miguel, M., Oliveira, R., Loureiro, N., García-Rubio, J. & Ibáñez, S. J. 2021. Load measures in Training/Match monitoring in soccer: A systematic review. *Int J Environ Res Public Health*, 18, 2721.

Myer, G. D., Ford, K. R., Brent, J. L. & Hewett, T. E. 2012. An integrated approach to change the outcome part II: Targeted neuromuscular training techniques to reduce identified ACL injury risk factors. *J Strength Cond Res*, 26, 2272–92.

Ostojic, S. M., Mazic, S. & Dikic, N. 2006. Profiling in basketball: Physical and physiological characteristics of elite players. *J Strength Cond Res*, 20, 2417–22.

Parsonage, J. R., Secomb, J. L., Tran, T. T., Farley, O. R. L., Nimphius, S., Lundgren, L. & Sheppard, J. M. 2017. Gender differences in physical performance characteristics of elite surfers. *J Strength Cond Res*, 31, 2417–22.

Portas, M. D., Harley, J. A., Barnes, C. A. & Rush, C. J. 2010. The validity and reliability of 1-Hz and 5-Hz global positioning systems for linear, multidirectional, and soccer-specific activities. *Int J Sports Physiol Perform*, 5, 448–58.

Randell, R. K., Clifford, T., Drust, B., Moss, S. L., Unnithan, V. B., De Ste Croix, M. B. A., Datson, N., Martin, D., Mayho, H., Carter, J. M. & Rollo, I. 2021. Physiological characteristics of female soccer players and health and performance considerations: A narrative review. *Sports Med (Auckland, N.Z.)*, 51, 1377–99.

Scott, M. T., Scott, T. J. & Kelly, V. G. 2016. The validity and reliability of global positioning systems in team sport: A brief review. *J Strength Cond Res*, 30, 1470–90.

Secomb, J. L., Farley, O. R. L., Lundgren, L., Tran, T. T., King, A. & Nimphius, S. 2015. Association between the performance of scoring manoeuvres and lower-body strength and power in elite surfers. *Int J Sports Sci Coach*, 10, 911–8.

Stojanović, E., Stojiljković, N., Scanlan, A. T., Dalbo, V. J., Berkelmans, D. M. & Milanović, Z. 2018. The activity demands and physiological responses encountered during basketball match-play: A systematic review. *Sports Med*, 48, 111–35.

Taylor, J. B., Ford, K. R., Nguyen, A.-D., Terry, L. N. & Hegedus, E. J. 2015. Prevention of lower extremity injuries in basketball: A systematic review and meta-analysis. *Sports Health*, 7, 392–8.

Tran, T. T., Lundgren, L., Secomb, J., Farley, O. R., Haff, G. G., Seitz, L. B., Newton, R. U., Nimphius, S. & Sheppard, J. M. 2015. Comparison of physical capacities between nonselected and selected elite male competitive surfers for the national junior team. *Int J Sports Physiol Perform*, 10, 178–82.

Trewin, J., Meylan, C., Varley, M. C. & Cronin, J. 2018. The match-to-match variation of match-running in elite female soccer. *J Sci Med Sport*, 21, 196–201.

Turner, A. N., Jones, B., Stewart, P., Bishop, C., Parmar, N., Chavda, S. & Read, P. 2019. Total score of athleticism: Holistic athlete profiling to enhance decision-making. *Strength Cond J*, 41, 91–101.

Vázquez-Guerrero, J., Suarez-Arrones, L., Casamichana Gómez, D. & Rodas, G. 2018. Comparing external total load, acceleration and deceleration outputs in elite basketball players across positions during match play. *Kinesiology*, 50, 228–34.

Vescovi, J. D. & Favero, T. G. 2014. Motion characteristics of women's college soccer matches: Female Athletes in Motion (FAiM) study. *Int J Sports Physiol Perform*, 9, 405–14.

Ziv, G. & Lidor, R. 2009. Physical attributes, physiological characteristics, on-court performances and nutritional strategies of female and male basketball players. *Sports Med*, 39, 547–68.

3   Injury Risk Assessment Including Flexibility

Joshua Miller

Part 1: Introduction – Movement Screen Testing

Muscular injury is one of the major problems facing professional and recreational athletes. Injuries to skeletal muscles account for more than 30% of the injuries seen by therapists and sports medicine physicians (NEISS, 2019). Nearly 2 million people each year in the United States suffer from sports-related injuries, ranging from relatively minor to quite serious (NEISS, 2019). These injuries are classified by the tissue that is injured. The different types of injuries include bone, muscle/tendon, joint, and spinal injuries (Amako et al. 2003; Garrett Jr. 1990; Armstrong 1990). Bone injuries are related to fractures. Muscle/tendon injuries are associated with sprains and strains. Joint injuries refer to the different types of joints in the body (i.e., ball-and-socket, sliding, and other types of joints). Finally, spinal injuries involve any type of injury to the spine, including the lower back. Injury risk assessment is the initial starting point for a strength and conditioning program to determine the individual's strengths and weaknesses to make sure the training program is created specifically for the athlete's requirements. The risk assessment results will expose weaknesses in the physical profile, which may predispose an athlete at risk for injury or limit performance. In addition, a coach knowing where the limits occur for a full ROM, especially during specific movement, will enable them to observe and address any issues immediately during training or practice.

Why Assess Injury Risk Assessment and Flexibility?

The aim of assessing injury risk by using a movement screening assessment allow to measure motor function and physical strength. The purpose of the movement screen is to identify how well an individual can complete basic and fundamental movement patterns. These movements are basic skills that support nearly every movement used in sport and life. Individuals that score poorly on these tests are unlikely to move well on the field, track, or any area that the individual participates in the sport they enjoy. The FMS requires flexibility, ROM, coordination, balance, and proprioception to complete the seven fundamental movement patterns (Cook et al., 2006a; Cook et al., 2006b). Upon completion of the screen, the results allow the individual to work with their strength and conditioning coach, physiotherapist, or physical therapist to improve their ability to move freely and efficiently, thus reducing the potential risk of injury in this individual.

The common reasons for injury by individuals are multifactorial. The common reasons for movements breaking down are due to lack of strength, ROM (mobility),

DOI: 10.4324/9781003186762-3

inability to control uninvolved joints (stability), and poor skill (motor control). Strength training has demonstrated a direct effect in preventing injuries, specifically hamstring muscle injuries. Walden et al. (2012) reported a 64% reduction in anterior cruciate ligament (ACL) injuries through improvement of core stability, pelvis control, and extremity coordination (Arendt, 2007; Steffen et al., 2010; Wilkerson and Colston 2015). Lauersen et al. (2014) reported that strength training was a better preventative than proprioception training and stretching in reduction of injuries. Lack of ROM is due to a joint being unable to move through a complete ROM during the assessment test. One such example would be seen performing a deep squat and the participants cannot lower themselves to the proper depth of thighs parallel with the ground; however, this can also be due to poor technique rather than limited. Issues with joint stability are demonstrated when muscles are unable to contract in the proper fashion to stabilize the joints. When the muscles are weakened, this may result in a poor movement pattern. Finally, poor skill is demonstrated when muscles do not relax and contract during appropriate times to allow the proper movement pattern to occur.

One of the most common movement screens that is conducted by coaches and therapists is the Functional Movement Screen® (FMS). The FMS has been utilized to determine potential risk of athletes, and non-athletes' risk of injury in multiple sports and military personnel (Kiesel et al., 2007; Miller and Susa, 2018; Chang et al., 2020; Davis, et al. 2020; Campa et al., 2019; Chapman et al. 2014; Lisman et al., 2018). The FMS places an individual in positions that will enable deficits to become noticeable if appropriate stability and mobility are not used. The athlete can complete fundamental movements using compensatory movements to achieve or maintain the level of performance required for the activity. The compensation leads to poor movement which can limit increases in performance and increases the risk of injury during training or sport. Researchers suggest that tests that assess multiple facets of function such as balance, strength, ROM, and motor control simultaneously may assist professionals in identifying athletes at risk for injury (Chorba et al., 2010; Kiesel et al., 2007; Plisky et al., 2006; Shimoura et al., 2019; Šiupsinkas et al., 2019). Thus the FMS does not evaluate the strength of the individual, rather allows to monitor changes in body movement. Total FMS scores have been investigated in relation to injury in National Football League (NFL) football players and in female collegiate soccer, basketball, and volleyball players (Kiesel et al., 2007; Chorba et al., 2010). Kiesel et al. (2007) reported an increase of 15% (pre-test probability) to 51% probability of football players sustaining a serious injury over the course of one season. It is estimated that there are between 18.4 and 5.17 injuries per 100 players (DeLee and Farney, 1992; Powell 1987). Chorba et al. (2010) found a significant correlation between low FMS scores (<14) in female athletes and lower extremity injury (in those without a prior ACL injury) participating in fall and winter sports. Furthermore, a score of 14 or less on the FMS resulted in an 11-fold increase in the risk of sustaining injury in professional football players and a 4-fold increase in the risk for lower extremity injury in female collegiate athletes (Kiesel et al., 2007; Chorba et al., 2010).

There are conflicting opinions reflecting methods of reducing injury through stretching which will increase flexibility or ROM. The coach's responsibility is to make sure an athlete can complete movements through a ROM or as completely as possible can determine if it will be necessary to make modifications to exercises that are being completed as part of their training program. Measuring ROM can be completed through sit-and-reach flexibility testing and goniometry. The sit-and-reach flexibility test includes the two muscle groups that have been suggested to be associated with low back pain – the hamstring and lower back muscles. The sit-and-reach test has been incorporated into several different national fitness battery tests such as the President's Council on Physical Fitness and Sports, the Fitnessgram, and AAHPERD Physical Best tests (Ref).

Part 2: Functional Movement Screen

The FMS consists of seven movement patterns that serve as a comprehensive functional movement. Additionally, four clearing tests, each associated with one of the FMS movement patterns, assess pain for the shoulder rotation motions, trunk extension, ankle flexion, and/or trunk flexion. An FMS kit can be purchased commercially (www.performbetter.com), but includes a 48-inch dowel rod, 2 smaller dowel rods approximately 24 inches, a 48-inch piece of 2″ × 6″ board, and an elastic band.

Testing should be completed in an open space that will allow for clearance of the dowel and movement of the individual in a minimum of an 8-foot area. The individual should be assessed in shorts and t-shirt or clothing that will enable complete visualization of the movements. All movements should be completed while wearing sneakers. When conducting the screening tests, athletes should not be bombarded with multiple instructions about how to perform the tests. Rather, the athlete should be moved to the starting position and then simple commands to allow for achievement of the test movement while observing performance. The coach will cue the athlete with the individual and clearing tests as they perform them to which may address balance, ROM, etc. The FMS is scored on a 4-point scale ranging from 0 to 3, where 3 is the best and 0 is the worst. An athlete is given a score of zero (0) if, at any time during the testing, they have any pain anywhere in the body. If pain occurs, a score of 0 is given and should be noted where the pain was located. A score of one (1) is given if the athlete is unable to complete the movement pattern or is unable to complete the movement. A score of two (2) is given when the athlete can complete the movement but compensates to perform the fundamental movement. A score of three (3) is given when the athlete performs the movement correctly without any compensation. The clearing tests are scored on a scale of positive or negative for pain only. If pain is present during the clearing test, then a score of 0 is placed for the score of that test.

The FMS consists of the following movements:

- Overhead squat
- In-line lunge
- Hurdle step
- Shoulder mobility
- Active straight-leg raise
- Trunk stability push-up
- Rotary stability test

There are four clearing tests that determine if the participant has any pain or limitations. These include the following movements:

- Ankle clearing after the in-line lunge test
- Shoulder clearing test after the shoulder mobility test

- Extension clearing test after the trunk stability push-up test
- Flexion clearing test after the rotary stability test

When testing the athlete observe from front and side views. All positions including foot position should remain unchanged throughout the test and score the test upon completion of complete movement. Do not coach the movement, repeat instructions as needed. Ask if the individual had any pain, and when in doubt, score low.

Testing Protocol of the Functional Movement Screen

1 **The Deep Squat**

   The deep squat assesses bilateral, symmetric mobility, and stability of the hips, knees, ankles, and core. The overhead position of the arms (holding the dowel) also assesses the mobility and symmetry of the shoulders and thoracic spine. To perform the test:

   i   The athlete starts with the feet at approximately shoulder width apart in the sagittal plane. Toes should be pointed forward throughout the test.
   ii   The dowel is grasped with both hands, and the arms are pressed overhead while keeping the dowel in line with the trunk and the elbows extended slightly wider than shoulder width.
   iii Arms will be a little wider than shoulder width.
   iv   The athlete is instructed to descend slowly and fully into a squat position while keeping the heels on the ground and the hands above the head.
   v   If unable to perform, athletes will be placed on the 48-inch 2″ × 6″ board with their heels on the board and the movement is repeated. This will be scored as a maximum of 2.
   vi   Score the test based upon completion of squat (Table 3.1, Figure 3.1).

2 **The Hurdle Step**

   The hurdle step is designed to challenge the ability to stride, balance, and perform a single-limb stance during coordinated movement of the lower extremity. To perform the test:

   i   The height of the hurdle or string should be equal to the height of the tibial tubercle of the athlete measured with the dowel rod.

Table 3.1 Scoring criteria for deep squat test.

Scoring Criteria = 3	Scoring Criteria = 2	Scoring Criteria = 1	Score Criteria = 0
• Upper torso is parallel with tibia or towards vertical • Femur below horizontal • Knees aligned over feet • Dowel aligned over feet	• Upper torso is parallel with tibia or toward vertical • Femur is below horizontal • Knees aligned over feet • Dowel aligned over feet on a 2 × 4	• Tibia and upper torso are not parallel • Femur not below horizontal • Knees not aligned over feet • Lumbar flexion noted	• Any pain at any time of movement

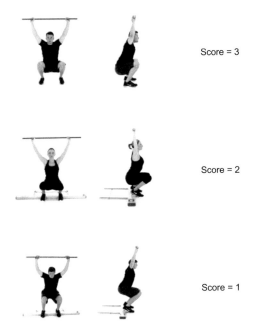

Figure 3.1 Examples of the different scores for the deep squat ranging between 1 and 3.

Note: Reprinted with the approval of the Functional Movement Screen.

ii Place the elastic band at the height of the tibial tuberosity.

iii The athlete assumes the start position by placing the feet together and aligning the toes just in contact with the base of the hurdle or 2 × 6 board (board will be placed on its side).

iv The dowel is placed across the shoulders below the neck, and the athlete is asked to step up and over the hurdle, touch the heel to the floor (without accepting weight) while maintaining the stance leg in an extended position, and return to the start position.

v The leg that is stepping over the hurdle is scored.

vi Repeat steps iii–v and score the opposite leg (Table 3.2, Figure 3.2).

Table 3.2 Scoring criteria for the Hurdle Step test.

Scoring Criteria = 3	*Scoring Criteria = 2*	*Scoring Criteria = 1*	*Score Criteria = 0*
• The hips, knees, and ankles remain aligned in the sagittal plane • Minimal movement in the lumbar spine • Dowel and hurdle remain parallel	• Alignment is lost between hips, knees, and ankles • Movement in the lumbar spine • Dowel and hurdle do not remain parallel	• Contact with foot and hurdle • Loss of balance at any time	• Any pain at any time of movement

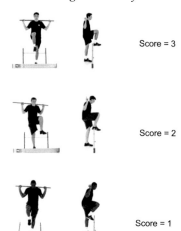

Score = 3

Score = 2

Score = 1

Figure 3.2 Examples of the different scores for the hurdle step.

Note: Reprinted with the approval of the Functional Movement Screen.

3 **In-Line Lunge**
   The in-line lunge attempts to challenge the athlete with a movement that challenges the athlete with balance and lateral challenge. To perform the test:

   i   Lunge length is determined by the tester by measuring the distance to the tibial tuberosity from the floor. (If not using an FMS kit: A piece of tape or a tape measure is placed on the floor at the determined lunge distance.)
   ii The arms are used to grasp the dowel behind the back with the top arm externally rotated, the bottom arm internally rotated, and the fists in contact with the neck and low back region.
   iii The hand opposite the front or lunging foot should be on top.
   iv The dowel must begin in contact with the thoracic spine, back of the head, and sacrum.
   v   The athlete is instructed to lunge out and place the heel of the front/lunge foot on the tape mark.
   vi The knee will touch the board momentarily.
   vii The athlete is then instructed to slowly lower the back knee enough to touch the floor while keeping the trunk erect and return to the start position.
   viii The front leg identifies the side being scored.
   ix Repeat steps ii–vii and score the opposite leg (Table 3.3, Figure 3.3).

Table 3.3 Scoring criteria for the in-line lunge.

Scoring Criteria = 3	Scoring Criteria = 2	Scoring Criteria = 1	Score Criteria = 0
• Minimal to no torso movement • Feet remain in sagittal plane of 2×6 • Knee touches 2×6 behind the heel of the front foot	• Movement noted in torso • Feet do not remain in sagittal plane on the 2×6 • Knee does not touch 2×6 behind the heel of front foot	• Loss of balance at any time	• Any pain at any time of movement

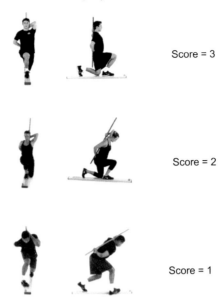

Score = 3

Score = 2

Score = 1

Figure 3.3 Examples of the different scores for the in-line lunge.

Note: Reprinted with the approval of the Functional Movement Screen.

Ankle Clearing Test

An important purpose for this clearing test is to identify pain and to ensure ankle mobility is not a barrier to the movement pattern. The lower body is adversely affected when ankle mobility is painful and/or limited. Normal, adequate mobility without pain is a prerequisite for movement patterns. To perform the test:

i   Place the outside of your left foot next to the test kit so that the outside foot is in contact with the kit.
ii Place the right foot in front of the left foot so that you are in the heel-to-toe position with both feet touching each other and the test kit and use a dowel for balance.
iii I will adjust the test kit so that the red start line is at the front of the medial malleolus.
iv While maintaining the heel-to-toe position, drop straight down, bending the back knee and taking it as far as possible in front of your toes while keeping the heel down.
v   Once you have reached your maximum distance, I will measure and ask you where you felt the stretch (front, back of ankle, or no stretch) (Table 3.4, Figure 3.4).

Table 3.4 Scoring criteria for the ankle clearing test.

Pass	Okay	Tight
• Knee moves beyond the medial malleolus of the front leg while the heel stays down • This indicates the ankle has cleared mobility requirements	• The knee resides within the width of the medial malleolus of the front leg while the heel stays down • This indicates a potential ankle mobility limitation	• The individual's knee does reach the medial malleolus of the front leg while the heel stays down • This indicates a potential ankle mobility limitation

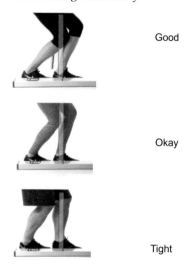

Good

Okay

Tight

Figure 3.4 Examples of the different scores for the ankle clearing test.

Note: Reprinted with the approval of the Functional Movement Screen.

Additional Considerations

- Pain: If the athlete experiences pain with this screen, indicate positive for pain in scoring and referral to a healthcare professional is recommended.
- Stretch: The goal of this ankle stretch is to be beyond 40 degrees of ankle dorsiflexion without ankle pain. However, if the athlete experiences a stretch or feeling of tightness of the ankle and it does not resolve with soft tissue or stretching applications, further assessment by a healthcare professional is needed. The excessive stretch or tightness should be above a normal feeling of discomfort associated with a static stretch.

4 Shoulder Mobility

This mobility screen assesses bilateral shoulder ROM by combining rotation and abduction/adduction motions. It also requires normal scapular and thoracic mobility. To perform the test:

i   Begin by determining the length of the hand of the athlete by measuring from the distal wrist crease to the tip of the third digit using the dowel rod. This distance is used during scoring of the test.

ii   The athlete is instructed to make a fist with each hand with the thumb placed inside the fist.

iii   The athlete is then asked to place both hands behind the back in a smooth motion (without walking or creeping them upward) – the upper arm in an externally rotated, abducted position (with a flexed elbow) and the bottom arm in an internally rotated, extended, and adducted position (also with a flexed elbow).

iv   The tester measures the distance between the 2 fists. The flexed (uppermost) arm identifies the side being scored.

v   Repeat and test the opposite arm following steps i–iv (Table 3.5, Figure 3.5).

Table 3.5 Scoring criteria for the shoulder mobility test.

Scoring Criteria = 3	Scoring Criteria = 2	Scoring Criteria = 1
• Fists should be within one hand length	• Fists should be within one-and-a-half hand lengths	• Fists fall greater than one-and-a-half hand lengths

Shoulder Clearing Test

After the shoulder mobility test is performed, the athlete places a hand on the opposite shoulder and attempts to point the elbow upward and touch the forehead. If painful, this clearing test is considered positive and the previous test must be scored as 0 (Figure 3.6).

5 **Active Straight-Leg Raise**

This test assesses the ability to move the lower extremity separately from the trunk, as well as tests for flexibility of the hamstring and gastrocnemius. To perform the test:

i   The athlete begins in a supine position, arms at the side.

ii   The tester identifies the midpoint between the anterior superior iliac spine and the middle of the patella and places a dowel on the ground, held perpendicular to the ground.

iii   The athlete is instructed to slowly lift the test leg with a dorsiflexed ankle and a straight knee as far as possible while keeping the opposite leg extended and in contact with the ground.

iv   Make note to see where the lower extremity ends at its maximal excursion. If the heel clears the dowel, a score of 3 is given; if the lower part of the leg

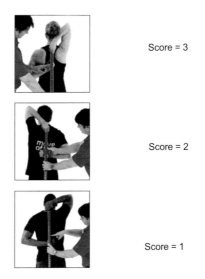

Score = 3

Score = 2

Score = 1

Figure 3.5 Examples of the different scores for the shoulder mobility test.

Note: Reprinted with the approval of the Functional Movement Screen.

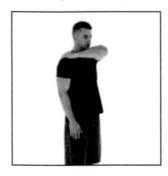

Figure 3.6 Example of the shoulder mobility clearing test.

Note: Reprinted with the approval of the Functional Movement Screen.

(between the foot and the knee) lines up with the dowel, a score of 2 is given; and if the patient is only able to have the thigh (between the knee and the hip) line up with the dowel, a score of 1 is given.

v   Repeat with the opposite leg (Table 3.6, Figure 3.7).

6   **Trunk Stability Push-up**
This test assesses the ability to stabilize the spine in anterior/posterior and sagittal planes during a closed-chain upper-body movement. To perform the test:

i   The athlete assumes a prone position with the feet together, toes in contact with the floor, and hands placed shoulder width apart (level determined by gender per criteria), as though ready to perform a push-up from the ground.

   a   For males – thumbs aligned with the forehead (score of 3), if unable to perform movement of thumbs to be aligned with the chin (maximal score of 2 possible)

   b   For females – thumbs are aligned with the chin (score of 3), if unable to perform movement of thumbs to be aligned with the clavicle (maximal score of 2 possible)

ii   The athlete is instructed to perform a single push-up in this position with the body lifted as a unit.

   a   If the athlete is unable to do this, the hands should be moved to a less-challenging position per criteria and a push-up attempted again as stated in step i(a) or i(b) based upon gender.

Table 3.6 Scoring criteria for the active straight leg test.

Scoring Criteria = 3	*Scoring Criteria = 2*	*Scoring Criteria = 1*	*Score Criteria = 0*
• Malleoli resides between mid-thigh and ASIS	• Malleoli resides between mid-thigh and mid-patella	• Malleoli resides below mid-patella	• Any pain at any time of movement

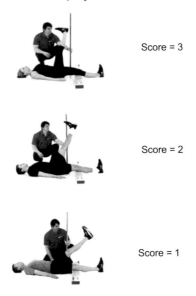

Score = 3

Score = 2

Score = 1

Figure 3.7 Examples of the different scores for the active-straight leg raise.

Note: Reprinted with the approval of the Functional Movement Screen.

 iii The chest and stomach should come off the floor at the same instance, and no "lag" should occur in the lumbar spine (Table 3.7, Figure 3.8).

Trunk Stability Push-Up Clearing Test

A clearing examination is performed at the end of the trunk stability push-up test and graded as pass or fail, failure occurring when pain is experienced during the test. Spinal extension is cleared by using a full-range prone press-up manoeuvre from the beginning push-up position; if pain is associated with this motion, a score of 0 is given (Figure 3.9).

 7 **Rotary Stability**

  The rotary stability test is a complex movement that requires neuromuscular control of the trunk and extremities and the ability to transfer energy between

Table 3.7 Scoring criteria for the Trunk Stability Push-up test.

Scoring Criteria = 3	*Scoring Criteria = 2*	*Scoring Criteria = 1*	*Score Criteria = 0*
• Males perform one repetition with the thumbs above head • Females perform one repetition with the thumbs in line with the chin	• Males perform one repetition with thumbs in line with the chin • Females perform one repetition with the thumbs in line with the clavicle	• Males unable to perform one repetition with hands in line with the chin • Females unable to perform one repetition with the hands in line with the clavicle	• Any pain at any time of movement

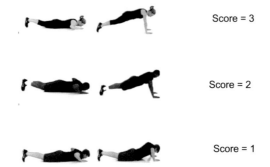

Score = 3

Score = 2

Score = 1

Figure 3.8 Examples of the different scores for the trunk stability push-up test.

Note: Reprinted with the approval of the Functional Movement Screen.

segments of the body. It assesses multiplane stability during a combined upper extremity and lower extremity motion. To perform the test:

   i The athlete will begin in a quadruped position, on their hands and knees, straddling the board with your thumbs, knees, and toes touching the board.

   ii Make sure the athlete's hands are under their shoulders and knees are under their hips with their feet pointing backward.

   iii At the same time, in one smooth and controlled motion, shift and lift the same side arm and leg.

   iv Without touching down, the athlete will reach back with their hand and touch the outside of the ankle.

   v Then extend that same side leg backward and arm forward, fully extending knee and elbow.

   vi Finally, reach back to touch the ankle with the hand again, and then return to the starting position.

   vii Perform this pattern while keeping the arm and leg moving in-line with the board.

   viii The test is repeated on the opposite side.

   ix The upper extremity that moves during testing is scored.

   x Completion of this task allows a score of 3. If unable to perform, the athlete is cued to perform the same manoeuvre with the opposite lower extremity and upper extremity, which allows a score of 2 to be awarded. Inability to perform a diagonal-touch stability results in a score of 1.

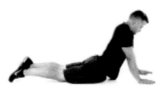

Figure 3.9 Example of the trunk stability push-up clearing test.

Note: Reprinted with the approval of the Functional Movement Screen.

Table 3.8 Scoring criteria for the trunk stability push-up test.

Scoring Criteria = 3	*Scoring Criteria = 2*	*Scoring Criteria = 1*	*Scoring Criteria = 0*
• Hand and knee leave ground at the same time • Ability to perform this pattern while keeping the arm and leg moving in-line and parallel with the board • Fingers touch the lateral malleolus • Knee and elbow achieve full extension	• Hand and knee did not leave ground at same time • Inability to keep the arm and leg moving in-line and parallel with the board • Fingers touch the lateral malleolus • Knee and elbow achieve full extension	• Loss of balance • Hand does not touch the lateral malleolus • Inability to get into starting position	• Any pain at any time of movement

xi   The test is then repeated for the opposite side and scored the same way using steps i–vi (Table 3.8, Figures 3.8 and 3.10).

Rotary Stability Clearing Test

A clearing examination is performed at the end of this test and again is scored as positive if pain is reproduced. From the beginning position for this test, the athlete rocks back into spinal flexion and touches the buttocks to the heels and the chest to the thighs. The hands should remain in contact with the ground. Pain on this clearing test overrides any score for the rotary stability test and causes the athlete to receive a score of 0 (Figure 3.11).

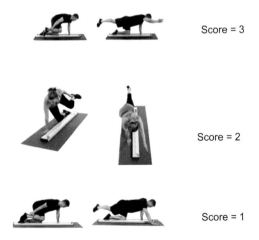

Score = 3

Score = 2

Score = 1

Figure 3.10 Examples of the different scores for the trunk stability push-up test.

Note: Reprinted with the approval of the Functional Movement Screen.

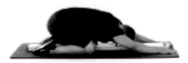

Figure 3.11 Example of the rotary stability clearing test.

Note: Reprinted with the approval of the Functional Movement Screen.

How to score the FMS

Score	Explanation
3	The person performs the movement correctly, without any compensation.
2	The person can complete the movement but must compensate in some way to complete the task.
1	The person is unable to complete the movement pattern or is unable to assume the position to perform the movement.
0	Any time during the test, the athlete has pain anywhere in the body. Clearing tests consider only pain, which would indicate a "positive" clearing test and requires a score of 0 for the test with which it is associated.

Data Interpretation for the Functional Movement Screen

A total score of 21 is the highest possible score on the FMS, which implies excellent and symmetric (in tests that are performed bilaterally) performance of the variety of screening manoeuvres (Figure 3.12).

1 **Raw Score:** This score is used when comparing movements for the individual sides right and left. Remember both sides are scored and are documented.
2 **Final Score:** This score is used for the overall score. When comparing right side with left side, the side that has the lower score will be used in the calculation of total score.
3 It is suggested that a score of less than 14 would be indicative of risk of injury. Previous studies have demonstrated a greater prevalence of athletes that have become injured either during the season or during training may be related to a lower FMS score (Kiesel et al., 2007; Chorba et al., 2010).

Movement Screen Test

1 **Overhead Squat**
This test will assess mobility of the thoracic spine, hips, and ankles, and determine the skill and control during a bilateral squat pattern.

Overhead Squat Procedures

i Grasp a dowel where the arms are wide enough to make 90° angles with the elbows and forearms.
ii Straighten the arms so that the broomstick is directly overhead.
iii Feet should be placed slightly wider than hip width with toes pointed slightly outwards.

Name: _____   Date: _____   DOB: _____

Height (cm): _____   Weight (kg): _____   Gender: _____

Distance from wrist to tip of finger: _____

Distance to patellar tendon: _____

Test	Raw Score	Final Score	Comments
Deep Squat			
Hurdle Step (L)			
Hurdle Step (R)			
Inline Lunge (L)			
Inline Lunge (R)			
Ankle Clearing Test			
Shoulder Mobility (L)			
Shoulder Mobility (R)			
Shoulder Clearing Test			
Active Straight Leg Raise (L)			
Active Straight Leg Raise (R)			
Trunk Stability Push-Up			
Push-up Clearing Test			
Rotary Stability (L)			
Rotary Stability (R)			
Rotary Clearing Test			
COMPOSITE SCORE			

Figure 3.12 Example of the scoring table for the Functional Movement Screen test.

    iv Lower into a squat by pushing the hips backwards and sitting through the heels.

    v Make sure the knees track over the toes and not to allow the feet move inward.

    vi The back should remain in a neutral position with the chest and head facing forward.

    vii Lower to a point just below parallel with the quadriceps or until the back is no longer in a neutral position.

    viii Return to the starting position and repeat two more times.

How to Score the Overhead Squat

Make sure to observe the movement from both the front and side while scoring (Yes and No only).

- Is the dowel or broomstick over the crown of the head?
- Is the low back in a neutral position?
- Did the quadriceps break parallel with the ground?
- Were the ankles able to stay on the ground?
- Did the knees track over the toes?

Typical errors that may be demonstrated during the overhead squat:

- Unable to maintain the dowel or broomstick over the crown of the head.
- Flexion in the lower back.
- Quadriceps do not break parallel with the ground
- Knees do not track over the toes.
- Ankles come off the ground during the lowering phase of the squat.

2 Single-Legged Hip Hinge

This test will assess the ability to hinge from the hips, determine the range of movement of the hamstrings, and also unilateral balance and control.

    i Stand with both feet on the ground and raise one foot off the ground.

    ii Slightly bend the knee of the support leg.

    iii Raise the arms out to the side to assist with balance.

    iv Contract the core musculature and raise the chest.

    v Bend at the hip while maintaining a straight support leg.

    vi Bend over until the torso is nearly parallel with the ground.

    vii Return to the starting position and repeat two more times.

How to Score the Single-Legged Hip Hinge

Make sure to observe the movement from both the front and side while scoring (Yes and No only):

- Is the lower back in a neutral position?
- Is the knee of the supporting leg only slightly bent?
- Did the participant move through a ROM that the torso is nearly parallel with the ground?
- Was each repetition performed with balance and control?

Typical errors that may be demonstrated during the single-legged hip hinge:

- Poor posture, i.e., inability to maintain a neutral lower back, unable to maintain a straight back

- Excessive bend in the support leg's knee
- Lack of ROM
- Misalignment of the shoulder-hip-ankle
- Lack of balance and control

3 **Standing Lunge**
This test will assess posture during a stepping movement, range of movement in hip extension, and unilateral balance and control:

 i   From a standing position with arms on hips and feet together, take a step forward, larger than a normal step so that the non-stepping foot's ankle is off the ground.
 ii Lower the hips towards the ground by bending at the knees.
 iii Descend so that the front leg quadricep is below parallel and the posterior knee nearly touches the ground.
 iv The torso should remain upright with the lower back in a neutral position.
 v   The posterior leg should be used for stabilization only.
 vi Return to the starting position and repeat two more times.

How to Score the Standing Lunge
Make sure to observe the movement from both the front and side while scoring (Yes and No only):

- Do the toes point forward, and is the weight of the posterior leg on the ball of the foot?
- Is there hip-knee-ankle alignment?
- Is the front foot aligned with knee over toes?
- Is the torso upright?
- Is the lower back in a neutral position and chest up?
- Is there balance and control?

Typical errors that may be demonstrated during the standing lunge:

- Rear foot flat on ground or twisted
- Front heel rise
- Hip-knee-ankle misalignment
- Torso not upright
- Poor posture
- Lack of balance and control

4 **Quadruped Superman**
This test will assess stability of the trunk and hips, and balance and control:

 i   Begin in a position with both hands and knees on the ground. Hands should be directly under the shoulders and knees directly under the hips.
 ii Back should be neutral and stabilize the core musculature.
 iii Slowly extend one arm to be parallel with the ground, while extending the opposite leg posteriorly.
 iv Bring the elbow of the extended arm and knee to touch in one movement without touching the ground with the hand or knee.
 v   Return to the starting position and repeat two more times.

How to Score the Quadruped Superman
Make sure to observe the movement from both the front and side while scoring (Yes and No only):

- Does the lower back remain in a neutral position at the end of the movement?
- Does the lower back remain in a neutral position when the knee and elbow touch?
- Does the movement remain stable so there is no movement to the right or left?
- Is there alignment with the shoulder-hip-ankle?
- Is there balance and control?

Typical errors that may be demonstrated during the quadruped superman:

- Unable to hold a neutral back.
- Shifting of the hips during the movement.
- Shoulder-hip-ankle misalignment.
- Lack of balance and control.

5 **Shoulder Mobility**
This test will assess bilateral shoulder ROM by combining rotation and abduction/adduction motions:

i   Begin by determining the length of the hand of the athlete by measuring from the distal wrist crease to the tip of the third digit using the dowel rod. This distance is used during scoring of the test.
ii The athlete is instructed to make a fist with each hand with the thumb placed inside the fist.
iii The athlete is then asked to place both hands behind the back in a smooth motion (without walking or creeping them upward) – the upper arm in an externally rotated, abducted position (with a flexed elbow) and the bottom arm in an internally rotated, extended, adducted position (also with a flexed elbow).
iv The tester measures the distance between the two fists. The flexed (uppermost) arm identifies the side being scored.
v   Repeat and test the opposite arm following steps ii–iv.

How to Score Shoulder Mobility
Make sure to observe the movement from both the front and side while scoring (Yes and No only):

- Is the movement smooth?
- Is the distance between the hands less than one-hand length?
- Is there any pain with the movement?

Typical errors that may be demonstrated during the quadruped superman:

- Inching the hands closer to one another behind the back?

Data Interpretation for the Functional Movement Screen

This movement screen utilizes a "Yes" or "No" answer scheme (Figure 3.13). There is no numerical scoring in comparison to the FMS test. The individuals that score poorly on these movements may move poorly on the field and are unable to complete complex movements during training. As a result, those individuals that have

Name: _____ Date: _____ DOB: _____

Height (cm): _____ Weight (kg): _____ Gender: _____

Make sure to observe the movement from both the front and side while scoring (Yes and No only).

Overhead Squat	Y/N	Single-leg Hip Hinge	Y/N	Standing Lunge	Y/N
Broomstick over head?		Lower back neutral?		Toes forward and on ball of rear foot?	
Lower back neutral?		Support leg slightly bent?		Hip-knee-ankle alignment?	
Quads break parallel?		Parallel to ground?		Torso upright?	
Ankles on ground?		Balance and control?		Lower back neutral?	
Knees over toes?				Balance and control?	

Quadruped Superman	Y/N	Shoulder Mobility	Y/N
Lower back neutral?		Movement smooth?	
Knee and elbow touch?		Distance < one-hand length?	
No extra movement?		Any pain?	
Should-hip-ankle alignment?			
Balance and control?			

Comments: _____

_____

_____

_____

Figure 3.13 Example of the scoring table for clearing test.

more "No" answers than "Yes" may be at greater risk of injury. Early screening and retraining proper movements may allow the coach or trainer to make adjustments and reduce the potential of injury in the future.

Part 2: Direct and Indirect Testing of Flexibility

Introduction

When measuring the ROM of a joint or a series of joints to determine a muscle's ability to lengthen within the limitation of the joint different techniques can be utilized in the lab. The measurement of the joint angle can be considered a direct measurement of flexibility. Flexibility is described as the ROM at a specific joint. An athlete can be very flexible at one joint but this does not mean that all joints will respond the same way. Therefore, there is not one test that can determine overall body flexibility. There are several different types of techniques that can be used to measure the ROM of a joint. This includes indirect and direct methods. One of the most common indirect methods for measuring flexibility is the sit-and-reach test. Direct methods for assessing flexibility measures the angular displacements between adjacent segments or from an external reference point is goniometry.

Indirect and direct methods use different tools to determine the ROM of a joint. A sit-and-reach box allows for the measurement of lower back flexibility to be determined in inches or centimetres where a goniometer determines ROM in degrees. With both methods, there are several variables that cannot be controlled during the test. For example, in the sit-and-reach test, the external zero point can be arbitrarily chosen or for goniometry, it may be difficult to identify the axis of motion for complex actions such as wrist flexion and extension which involve more than two bony articulations (Moore, 1948).

Direct Technique: Goniometry

The goniometer is a protractor-like device with two steel or plastic arms that measure the joint angle at different ROM (see Figure 3.14) and will be used to measure the ROM at a joint in degrees. There are different types of goniometers that can be used to measure ROM. Digital goniometers provide a digital ROM value rather than having to read the value off the device itself by the practitioner. Carey et al. (2010) reported no significant differences between universal and digital goniometers when measuring joint ROM, and the inter- and intrarater reliability is equivalent to the universal goniometer. The digital goniometer may reduce reader errors when reading the value from the screen in comparison to the universal device.

The stationary arm of the goniometer is attached at the zero line of the protractor, and the other arm is moveable. To use the goniometer, place the centre of the device so it coincides with the axis of rotation of the joint. Align the arms of the goniometer with the bony landmarks along the longitudinal axis of each moving body segment. Measure the ROM as the difference between the joint angles (degrees) from the beginning to the end of the movement. Table 3.9 describes goniometer measurement for various joints.

Once measurements of various joint ROMs have been completed, comparison can be made with healthy adults. Table 3.10 presents average ROM value for healthy adults.

When utilizing goniometry, ROM can be determined to determine if the joint can move through a complete ROM to determine if there may be an underlying issue associated with injury or structural abnormality.

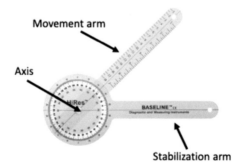

Figure 3.14 A goniometer, including the body axis or fulcrum, a stabilization arm, and movement.

Table 3.9 Average range of motion (ROM) for different joints in healthy adults.

Joint	ROM (degrees)	Joint	ROM (degrees)
Shoulder		Thoracic-Lumbar spine	
Flexion	150–180	Flexion	60–80
Extension	50–60	Extension	20–30
Abduction	180	Abduction	25–35
Medial rotation	70–90	Rotation	30–45
Lateral rotation	90	Hip	
Elbow		Flexion	100–120
Flexion	140–150	Extension	30
Extension	0	Abduction	40–45
Radioulnar		Adduction	20–30
Pronation	80	Medial Rotation	40–45
Supination	80	Lateral Rotation	45–50
Wrist		Knee	
Flexion	60–80	Flexion	135–150
Extension	60–80	Extension	0
Radial Deviation	20	Ankle	
Ulnar Deviation	30	Dorsiflexion	20
Cervical Spine		Plantar Flexion	40–45
Flexion	45–60	Subtalar	
Extension	45–75	Inversion	30–35
Lateral Flexion	45	Eversion	15–20
Rotation	60–80		

Case Study

A coach wants to measure the ROM of their athlete's hip flexion utilizing the Hamstring Criterion Test. To perform the test, the athletes will lay on their back on a plinth or bench. The goniometer is placed at the athlete's hip joint. The stationary arm is placed in line with the trunk and the moving arm in line with the femur. The athlete's knee will be straight while moving the leg towards hip flexion. Once

Table 3.10 Age-gender norms for the standard sit-and-reach test.

	15–19 years	20–29 years	30–39 years	40–49 years	50–59 years	60–69 years
Men						
Excellent	≥ 39	≥ 40	≥38	≥ 35	≥ 35	≥ 33
Very good	34–38	34–39	33–37	29–34	28–34	25–32
Good	29–33	30–33	28–32	24–28	24–27	20–24
Fair	24–28	25–29	23–27	18–23	16–23	15–19
Needs improvement	≤ 23	≥ 24	≥ 22	≥ 17	≥ 15	≥ 14
Women						
Excellent	≥ 43	≥ 41	≥ 41	≥ 38	≥ 39	≥ 35
Very good	38–42	37–40	36–40	34–37	33–38	31–34
Good	34–37	33–36	32–35	30–33	30–32	27–30
Fair	29–33	28–32	27–31	25–29	25–29	23–26
Needs improvement	≥ 28	≥ 27	≥ 26	≥ 24	≥ 24	≥ 22

Data adapted from Greene and Heckman (1994) and Levangie, Norkin and Lewek (2019).

Distance is measured in centimetres.

tightness is felt by the coach, the leg is helped there and the ROM is read from the goniometer. The test is repeated two additional times. The measurements were 112°, 115°, and 110°. The measurement is averaged and compared to the normative data for hip flexion (0–120°). The results would fall within normal limits.

Indirect Technique (Sit-and-reach)

Indirect measurement of static flexibility can be determined with the use of a sit-and-reach test. This test is one of the most common health-related fitness tests that is used to evaluate static flexibility of the lower back and hamstring muscles (Payne et al., 2000). The sit-and-reach test provides an indirect measurement of the ROM. There are several different types of sit-and-reach tests that have been developed using a box, yardstick, or both to measure flexibility in inches or centimetres. Several studies have demonstrated that the sit-and-reach test is moderately related to hamstring flexibility (r = .46–.67), but poorly related to low back flexibility (r = .16–.35) in adults (Mayorga-Vega et al., 2014) and in older adults independently living (r = .54–.74) (Lemmink et al., 2003).

Methodological Information

There are several different protocols for various sit-and-reach tests. Prior to having the athlete complete the protocol, have them perform a general warm-up to increase muscle temperature, as well as hamstring and lower back stretches. The athlete's shoes should be removed for all the different protocols.

1   **Standard Sit-and-Reach Test**
    This test utilizes a sit-and-reach box (Figure 3.14) with a zero point at 26 cm. To perform the test:

    i   The athletes will sit on the floor with their knees extended and the soles of their feet against the edge of the box.
    ii   The feet must be 6 in. (15.2 cm) apart.
    iii Remind the athletes to keep their knees fully extended, arms evenly stretched, and hands placed on top of one another with their palms down as they slowly reach forward as far as possible along the top of the box.
    iv   Have the athlete lower their head between their extended arms while exhaling throughout the movement.
    v   Hold this position for approximately 2 seconds and then have them return to the starting position.
    vi   Repeat the test twice and record the highest test to the nearest 0.5 cm as the maximal score.
    vii Report data on sheet (Figure 3.15).

    Remind the athletes not to bend their knees or perform the movement in a bouncing or jerky movement. If they do, have them repeat the trial. Repeat the test twice and record the highest test to the nearest 0.5 cm as the maximal score. Tables 3.11–3.13 present age–gender norms for this test from males, females, and sport-specific athletes.

Name: _____ Date: _____ DOB: _____

Height (cm): _____ Weight (kg): _____ Gender: _____

Type of Sit-and-Reach Test: _____

	Trial 1	Trial 2	Trial 3
Distance (in.)			

Greatest Distance (in.):_____

Classification: _____

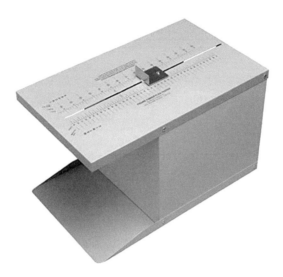

Figure 3.15 Example of the scoring table for the Sit-and-Reach test.

2 V Sit-and-Reach Test

The V sit-and-reach test, or the YMCA test (YMCA, 2000), uses a yardstick instead of a box. Prior to testing, make sure the yardstick is secured to the floor by placing tape at the 15-in. (38-cm) mark on the yardstick. To perform the test:

i   The athletes will sit, straddling the yardstick, with their knees extended (but not locked out), and their feet 12 in. (30.5 cm) apart.
ii   The heels of their feet should be touching the 15-in. mark.
iii   Make sure their knees do not flex and they do not extend one arm further than the other one.
iv   Have the athlete lower their head between their extended arms while exhaling throughout the movement.
v   Hold this position for approximately 2 seconds and then have them return to the starting position.
vi   Repeat the test twice and record the highest test to the nearest 0.5 cm as the maximal score.

Table 3.11 Percentile ranks for the modified sit-and-reach test in females.

	Females			
	< 18 years	19–35 years	36–49 years	> 50 years
Percentile rank				
99	57.4	53.3	50.3	43.7
95	49.5	49.0	48.8	39.9
90	47.5	45.5	44.2	38.1
80	45.2	42.4	41.1	36.1
70	41.9	41.1	38.6	34.5
60	40.6	40.1	36.8	31.2
50	38.6	37.6	34.3	28.2
40	36.8	36.8	32.5	25.7
30	34.8	34.8	31.0	23.4
20	32.0	32.0	27.9	21.1
10	29.0	25.7	24.6	19.1

Distance is measured in centimetres.

Remind the athletes not to bend their knees or perform the movement in a bouncing or jerky movement. If they do, have them repeat the trial. Repeat the test twice and record the highest test to the nearest 0.5 cm as the maximal score.

3   **Back-Saver Sit-and-Reach Test**
The Back-Saver test was created to relieve some of the discomfort of the lower back when compared to the standard, modified, and V sit-and-reach tests. The validity of the version of the sit-and-reach test is very similar to the standard version in men ($r = .47$–.67) and in women ($r = .023$–0.54) (Hui and Yuen 2000). This test measures the flexibility of the hamstrings one leg at a time. To perform the test:

i   Tell the athlete to place the sole of the extended foot against the edge of the sit-and-reach box.

Table 3.12 Percentile ranks for the modified sit-and-reach test in males.

	Males			
	< 18 years	19–35 years	36–49 years	> 50 years
Percentile rank				
99	51.7	62.7	48.0	41.1
95	49.8	48.0	46.2	40.1
90	46.2	43.7	40.9	38.1
80	45.2	43.2	37.1	33.8
70	40.6	40.1	35.3	31.2
60	38.6	38.1	34.0	29.2
50	36.8	36.6	32.0	25.9
40	35.6	34.3	29.5	24.6
30	34.0	33.0	27.4	23.6
20	30.0	29.5	25.1	22.4
10	24.1	23.4	21.1	19.8

Distance is measured in centimetres.

Table 3.13 Mean and standard deviation of the Sit-and-Reach test in athletes.

Sport	Level	Gender	Age	Sit-and-reach	Reference
Volleyball	NCAA Division I	F	19.6 (0.6)	17.3 (4.9)	Fry et al. (1991)
Basketball	Professional	M			Parr et al. (1978)
C	NBA		27.7 (5.2)	14.8 (0.0)	
F			25.3 (3.8)	16.2 (2.7)	
G			25.2 (3.6)	15.9 (3.1)	
Football	NCAA	M			Schmidt (1999)
DB	Division III		19.9 (1.4)	11.4 (3.8)	
L			19.9 (1.6)	14.2 (5.2)	
TE/LB			19.9 (1.2)	10.5 (6.5)	
Football	NCAA	M			Stuempfle et al. (2003)
Team	Division III		19.6 (1.3)	12.1 (5.9)	
OL			19.0 (1.1)	10.7 (3.9)	
DL			19.5 (1.2)	14.3 (6.1)	
OB			19.9 (1.4)	11.4 (6.4)	
DB			19.8 (1.2)	12.1 (5.9)	

Data is reported in centimetres.

C = centre; F = forward, G = guard; DB = defensive back; L = lineman; TE = tight end; LB = linebacker; OL = offensive lineman; DL = defensive lineman; OB = offensive back.

ii Flex the untested leg by placing the sole of the foot flat on the floor 2–3 in. (5–8 cm) to the side of the extended knee.

iii Follow the same directions of the standard sit-and-reach test.

iv Repeat the test for the opposite leg.

Data Interpretation

Table 3.13 demonstrates different mean and standard deviations for different competitive sports in high school, college, and professional sports.

Laboratory Task: Are You at Risk of Injury?

• Complete different types of measurements on risk for injury and flexibility.

Summary

Physical inactivity is a major cause of inflexibility and can lead to injuries. Injury prevention is the key to longevity of the athlete's career whether they are a professional or recreational athlete. Using the Functional Movement Screen to determine potential risk of injury as well muscle imbalances can direct training programs to reduce this possible risk. Flexibility is highly joint specific and the ROM, partly, depends upon the structure of the joint. Incorporating indirect and/or direct measurements of flexibility can ensure proper mobility of a joint. Goniometry allows for a direct measurement, whereas the Sit-and-Reach test uses indirect assessment of the ROM of the specific joints.

References

Amako, M., Oda, T., Masuoka, K., Yokoi, H. & Campisi, P. 2003. Effect of static stretching on prevention of injuries for military recruits. *Mil Med*, 168, 442–6.

Arendt, E. 2007. Core strengthening. *Instr Course Lec*, 56, 379–84.

Armstrong, B. A., 1990. Initial events in exercise-induced muscular injury. *Med Sci Sports Exerc*, 22, 429–35.

Campa, F., Piras, F., Raffi, M. & Toselli, S. 2019. Functional movement patterns and body composition of high-level volleyball, soccer, and rugby players. *J Sport Rehabil*, 28, 740–5.

Carey, M. A., Laird, D. E., Murray, K. A. & Stevenson, J. R. 2010. Reliability, validity, and clinical usability of a digital goniometer. *Work*, 36, 55–66.

Chang, W. D., Chou, L. W., Chang, N. J. & Chen, S. 2020. Comparison of functional movement screen, star excursion balance test, and physical fitness in junior athletes with different sports injury risk. *Biomed Res Int*, 25, 2020:8690540.

Chapman, R. F., Laymon, A.S. & Arnold, T. 2014. Functional movement scores and longitudinal performance outcomes in elite track and field athletes. *Int J Sports Physiol Perform*, 9, 203–11.

Chorba, R. S., Chorba, D. J., Bouillon, L. E., Overmyer, C. A. & Landis, J. A. 2010. Use of a functional movement screening tool to determine injury risk in female collegiate athletes. *N Am J Sports Phys Ther*, 5, 47–54.

Cook, G., Burton, L. & Hogenboom, B. 2006a. The use of fundamental movements as an assessment of function – Part 1. *NAJSPT*, 1, 62–72.

Cook, G., Burton, L. & Hogenboom, B. 2006b. Pre-participation screening: The use of fundamental movements as an assessment of function – Part 2. *NAJSPT*, 1, 132–9.

Davis, J. D., Orr, R., Knapik, J. J. & Harris, D. 2020. Functional Movement Screen (FMS™) scores and demographics of US Army pre-ranger candidates. *Mil Med*, 185, e788–94.

DeLee, J. C. & Farney, W. C. 1992. Incidence of injury in Texas high school football. *Am J Sports Med*, 20, 575–80.

Fry, A. C., Kraemer, W. J., Weseman, C. A., Conroy, B. P., Gordon, S. E., Hoffman, J. R. & Maresh, C. M. 1991. The effects of off-season strength and conditioning program on starters and non-starters in women's intercollegiate volleyball. *J Strength Cond Res*, 5, 174–81.

Garrett, Jr., W. E. 1990. Muscle strain injuries: Clinical and basic aspects. *Med Sci Sports Exerc*, 22, 436–43.

Greene, W. B. & Heckman, J. D. 1994. *The Clinical Measurement of Joint Motion*. Rosemont, IL: American Academy of Orthopedic Surgeons.

Hui, S. S. & Yuen, P. Y. 2000. Validity of the modified back-saver sit-and-reach test: a comparison with other protocols. *Med Sci Sports Exerc*, 32, 1655–9.

Kiesel, K. Plisky, P. J. & Voight, M. L. 2007. Can serious injury in professional football be predicted by a preseason functional movement screen? *N Am J Sports Phys Ther*, 2, 147–52.

Lauersen, J. B., Bertelsen, D. M. & Andersen, L. B. 2014. The effectiveness of exercise interventions to prevent sport injuries: A systematic review and meta-analysis of randomized controlled studies. *Br J Sports Med*, 48, 871–7.

Lemmink, K. A., Kemper, K. A., de Greef, M. H., Rispens, P. & Stevens, M. 2003. The validity of the sit-and-reach test and the modified sit-and-reach test in middle-aged to older men and women. *Res Q Exerc Sport*, 74, 331–6.

Levangie, P. K., Norkin, C. C. & Lewek M. D. 2019. *Joint Structure and Function*. 6th ed. Philadelphia, PA: FA Davis Company, 552.

Lisman, P., Nadelen, M., Hildebrand, E., Leppert, K. & de la Motte, S. 2018. Functional movement screen and Y-balance test scores across levels of American football players. *Biol Sport*. 35, 253–60.

Mayorga-Vega, D., Merino-Marban, R. & Viciana, J. 2014. Criterion-related validity of sit-and-reach tests for estimating hamstring and lumbar extensibility: A meta-analysis. *J Sports Sci Med*, 13, 1–14.

Miller, J. M. & Susa, K. J. 2018. Functional movement screen in a group of division IA athletes. *J Sports Med Phys Fitness*, 59, 779–83.

Moore, M. L. (1948). The measurement of joint motion; the technic of goniometry. *Phys Ther Rev*, 29, 256-264.

NEISS. 2019. Data Highlights – 2019. *Consumer Product Safety Commission (CPSC)*, Bethesda, MD.

Parr, R. B., Hoover, R., Wilmore, J. H., Bachman, D. & Kerlan, R. K. 1978. Professional Basketball Players: Athletic Profiles. *Phys Sportsmed*, 6, 77–87.

Payne, N. Gledhill, N., Katzmarzyk, P. T., Jamnik, V. K. & Keir, P. J. 2000. Canadian musculoskeletal fitness norms. *Can J Appl Physiol*, 25, 430–42.

Plisky, P. J., Rauh, M. J., Kaminski, T. W. & Underwood, F. B. 2006. Star excursion balance test as a predictor of lower extremity injury in high school basketball players. *J Orthop Sports Phys Ther*, 36, 911–9.

Powell, J. 1987. Incidence of injury associated with playing surfaces in the national football league. *J Alth Train*, 22, 202–6.

Schmidt, W. D. 1999. Strength and physiological characteristics of NCAA Division III American football players. *J Strength Cond Res*, 13, 210–3.

Shimoura, K., Nakayama, Y., Tashiro, Y., Hotta, T., Suzuki, Y., Tasaka, S., Matsushita, K., Kawagoe, M., Sonoda, T., Yokota, Y. & Aoyama, T. 2019. Association between functional movement screen scores and injuries in male college basketball players. *J Sport Rehabil*, 29, 621–5.

Šiupšinkas, L., Garbenyte-Apolinskiene, T., Salakaite, S., Gudas, R. & Trumpockas, V. 2019. Association of pre-season musculoskeletal screening and functional testing with sports injuries in elite female basketball players. *Sci Rep*, 9, 9286.

Steffen, K., Andersen, T. E., Krosshaug, T., et al. 2010. ECCS Position Statement 2009: Prevention of acute sports injuries. *Eur J Sport Sci*, 10, 223–36.

Stuempfle, K. J., Katch, F. I. & Petrie, D. F. 2003. Body composition relates poorly to performance tests in NCAA Division III football players. *J Strength Cond Res*, 17, 238–44.

Walden, M., Atroshi, I., Magnusson, H., et al. 2012. Prevention of acute knee injuries in adolescent female football players: cluster randomised control trial. *BMJ*, 344, e3042.

Wilkerson, G. B. & Colston, M. A. 2015. A refined prediction model for core and lower extremity sprains and strains among collegiate football players. *J Athl Train*, 50, 643–50.

YMCA of the USA. 2000. *YMCA Fitness Testing and Assessment Manual*, 4th ed. Champaign, IL: Human Kinetics.

4 Statistical Analysis and Test Administration

John McMahon, Joshua Miller, and Paul Comfort

Part 1: Introduction

As described in detail in Chapter 2, strength and conditioning coaches will likely assess their athletes' physical capabilities in a variety of ways depending upon the nature of the sport (as determined following the completion of a thorough needs analysis). The tests used to physically assess athletes will likely involve a variety of measurement devices and will either require the strength and conditioning coach to conduct their own data analyses to extract key metrics of interest (such as sprint speed from a timing device [see Chapter 11], for example) or this will be done via the software associated with the measurement device (e.g., automated force plate systems). In the case of the latter scenario, we encourage strength and conditioning coaches to ask software manufacturers how their calculations are performed to facilitate comparisons with published data or those obtained from an equivalent device by another company (i.e., a different brand). In either case, strength and conditioning coaches should ascertain the reliability, measurement error and, whenever possible, the validity of the metrics obtained by the test devices that they use to allow them to interpret the data more effectively and thus better apply it to their athletes' training program design.

Part 2: Reliability

Intraclass Correlation Coefficient

A test of reliability should consider both the degree of correlation and the agreement between measurements (Koo and Li, 2016). The suggested statistical test for this purpose is the intraclass correlation coefficient (ICC) (Shrout and Fleiss, 1979). There are ten forms of ICC which differ based on "model," "type," and "definition" selections and the precise form required will depend on the intended application (Koo and Li, 2016). Most strength and conditioning coaches will be interested in applying the ICC to determine the test-retest reliability of chosen test metrics, such as the vertical jump height obtained during a countermovement jump, for example. In this case, a two-way mixed effects ICC "model" should be selected (Koo and Li, 2016). Then a decision must be made to which "type" of ICC should be selected and this depends on whether the data represent a single measurement or the mean average of multiple measurements (Koo and Li, 2016). For example, several researchers have suggested that the average across two or more countermovement jump trials should be taken forward for statistical analyses rather than the single best trial (which is usually decided as the trial which

DOI: 10.4324/9781003186762-4

led to the highest jump) (Kennedy and Drake, 2021; Claudino et al., 2017). Thus, we recommend that strength and conditioning coaches should utilize the mean average of multiple (often denoted by a k) for test-retest applications. Finally, based on these ICC "model" and "type" decisions, the absolute agreement ICC "definition" should be applied (Koo and Li, 2016). The maximum value that any form of ICC can be is 1 and in simple terms, the closer to 1, the more reliable the test. However, the data should be interpreted based on the representative spread of the ICC, based on the lower bound 95% confident interval (CI) of the estimated ICC value, <0.50, between 0.50 and 0.75, between 0.75 and 0.90, and >0.90 are indicative of poor, moderate, good, and excellent reliability, respectively (Koo and Li, 2016). When the lower- and upper-bound 95% CIs of the ICC estimate are wide, the range of qualitative interpretations that they span should be acknowledged. For example, if the estimated ICC is 0.80, and the lower- and upper-bound 95% CIs are 0.65 and 0.95, respectively, the interpretation should be that the reliability was "moderate to excellent" rather than "good," as the estimated ICC value of 0.80 alone would suggest.

Recommendations for determining a sufficient sample size when applying the ICC to test-retest study designs were recently published (Borg et al., 2022). Given that most strength and conditioning coaches work with limited athlete numbers, they may struggle to conduct test-retest reliability analyses within single squads. One solution to this might be to group athletes of a similar age and/or ability together to reach a large enough sample size. In any case, low sample sizes can lead to erroneous ICC values (Borg et al., 2022) and so they should be avoided where possible. Based on the sample size lookup tables provided by Borg et al. (2022), researchers and practitioners can estimate the minimum sample size required depending on whether the goal is to estimate the desired ICC with sufficient precision, based on an estimation approach, or to demonstrate that the ICC is above a particular threshold, e.g., higher than 0.75 (i.e., the threshold for "good" reliability according to Koo and Li, 2016), based on a hypothesis testing approach. The hypothesis testing approach is usually applied within strength and conditioning research settings and normally a test-retest study design would only include two testing sessions (e.g., day 1 and day 2, as shown in Figure 4.1). Based on these assumptions, an estimation of the anticipated ICC value (which can be based on ICC values reported in published studies) and a minimum statistical power requirement of either 80% (most typical) or 90%, the minimum sample size requirement can be estimated (Borg et al., 2022). Let's say we plan to conduct a test-retest study involving the countermovement jump test over two sessions separated by one week and we want the ICC for vertical jump height to be above 0.75 to be considered good (Koo and Li, 2016), and we anticipate the test-retest ICC for vertical jump height in the countermovement jump test to be 0.90 based on a published study (McMahon et al., 2018), and we want a minimal statistical power of 80%. In this scenario, the minimum sample size recommendation is 33, according to Borg et al. (2022). This minimum sample size should be achievable for many strength and conditioning coaches who work in team sports by involving two squads of a similar age and ability (e.g., the under-16s and under-18s in a soccer club).

As visually shown in Figure 4.1, an excellent ICC value is observed when athletes achieve the same rank for the test metric on each test occasion (shown in the left panel of Figure 4.1). Thus, the more that athletes switch ranks on each test occasion, the worse the ICC for the test metric will be. In the right panel of Figure 4.1, for example, the best performing athlete who attained a jump height of 54 cm on day 1 was

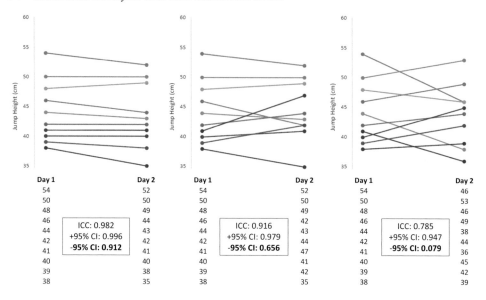

Figure 4.1 Example of excellent (left panel), moderate (middle panel), and poor (right panel) test-retest intraclass correlation coefficient (ICC) results according to the lower bound 95% confidence interval (CI) which is highlighted in bold text. The jump height data (in cm) used to create each figure is shown below them.

the joint-third performing athlete with a jump height of 46 cm on day 2. Similarly, the lowest scoring athlete for jump height on day 1 (jump height = 38 cm) was third from bottom on day 2 (jump height = 45 cm). Therefore, a test metric that has a poorer ability to rank athletes' performances will yield a lower ICC value and so will be considered to have poorer relative reliability compared to a test that does well at distinguishing athlete performance levels.

It is important to note that the familiarity of the athlete with the test will influence the resultant ICC values. Thus, strength and conditioning coaches should allow their athletes to become acquainted with a test before having confidence in the results. Also, working with homogenous groups, as is common when working with athletes, may negatively affect the ICC due to the potentially reduced spread of scores across the group. There can be instances where the relative reliability is high, thus the test metric assessed can distinguish well between athletes between trials or test occasions (depending on the application), but the absolute reliability is low. That is why it is also important to assess the absolute reliability (i.e., measurement error) for key measurements, particularly if being used to monitor changes over time.

Standard Error of Measurement

The most common statistical test used to assess absolute reliability is the standard error of measurement (SEM) which is most often reported as a coefficient of variation (CV) expressed as a percentage of the observed mean value. The measurement error of a test metric will vary from athlete to athlete, independently of magnitude of the score obtained so it cannot be predicted. Thus, we must estimate the average measurement error for a cohort by estimating the within-athlete variability and assuming that it is the same for all athletes, which is an accepted limitation of this approach. The SEM calculation may not always be embedded in common statistical analysis packages but can easily be calculated in common applications such as Microsoft Excel (Figure 4.2). To calculate the SEM, firstly the difference score between the two testing occasions (e.g., day 1 and day 2) can be calculated for each athlete by subtracting their session 1 mean score from their session 2 mean score for each test metric. Each athlete's mean score obtained for each session is calculated as the mean (i.e., average) score across the trials recorded for each test (e.g., the average of three trials, if that is how many trials the athletes did). The between-athlete standard deviation of the difference scores for each test metric can then be calculated and the answer divided by the square root of 2 to give the SEM (Swinton et al., 2018). This method of calculating the SEM is said to be numerically equivalent to the "direct method" when we have just two measurements for each participant (or two session average measurements, as is the case in the example described thus far and, in most applied sports environments). The 95% CI of the SEM can be calculated by multiplying it by 1.96. Both the SEM and SEM + 95% CI can be expressed as a CV percentage by dividing them by the grand mean (the between-athlete mean score across sessions 1 and 2) and multiplying the answer by 100. The minimal detectible change (MDC) can be calculated by multiplying the SEM + 95% CI by the square root of 2 (see Figure 4.2). The MDC can also be expressed as a percentage by dividing it by the grand mean and multiplying the answer by 100.

Each of the calculations explained above is shown in Figure 4.2 and is applied to countermovement jump height data that are also presented in Figure 4.1 (left panel). Based on these data, the strength and conditioning coach could assume that (1) 95% of countermovement jump height measurements will fall within 1.7 cm of what is

▲	A	B	C	D	E	F
1		Athlete Number	JH Day 1 (cm)	JH Day 2 (cm)	Difference Score (cm)	
2		1	54	52	2	
3		2	50	50	0	
4		3	48	49	-1	
5		4	46	44	2	
6		5	44	43	1	
7		6	42	42	0	
8		7	41	41	0	
9		8	40	40	0	
10		9	39	38	1	
11		10	38	35	3	
12		Mean	44.2	43.4	0.8	
13						
14					Formula:	
15			SD of Diffs (cm)	1.2	=STDEV(E2:E11)	
16			SEM (cm)	0.9	=D15/SQRT(2)	
17			SEM +95% CI (cm)	1.7	=D16*1.96	
18			Grand Mean (cm)	43.8	=AVERAGE(C12:D12)	
19			SEM CV (%)	2.0	=(D16/D18)*100	
20			MDC (cm)	2.4	=D17*SQRT(2)	

Figure 4.2 An example of how to calculate absolute reliability in Microsoft Excel with formulae shown. JH = jump height; SD = standard deviation; Diffs = differences; SEM = standard error or measurement; CI = confidence interval; CV = coefficient of variation; MDC = minimal detectible change.

observed for an athlete who is from a similar cohort and (2) 2.4 cm is the minimal amount of change in countermovement jump height required to exceed measurement error. These assumptions are based on the athletes being from the same sport, from a similar competitive level and tested using equivalent methods (e.g., same instrumentation [e.g., force plate] and jump height calculation [e.g., from impulse-momentum theorem]). This information is useful to strength and conditioning coaches as it promotes caution when interpreting data obtained from testing their athletes. We should remember that due to both instrumentation and biological noise (i.e., unwanted disturbance in an electrical signal) being present whenever we test our athletes (Swinton et al., 2018), we cannot know what an athlete's "true" test score is and, therefore, what a true change in the test score is. Instead, we should interpret the observed data for our athletes alongside the SEM +95% CI and MDC each time we assess them.

Concurrent Validity

There are many types of validity, but concurrent validity is arguably of most relevance to strength and conditioning coaches in the context of physically testing athletes. Concurrent validity specifies the amount of agreement between two different test devices that purportedly measure the same thing (Adams et al., 2014). As strength and conditioning coaches, we should attempt to test our athletes with devices that have been concurrently validated against an assumed criterion device (i.e., an industry gold standard) wherever possible to give us and our athletes' confidence in the data. The concurrent validity of a new test device should be determined by quantifying the agreement between it and a well-established test device that has already been proven (or is considered) to be valid (i.e., a criterion device). It should be noted that a test device can be reliable but not valid. For example, some electronic contact mats that are commonly used to test an athlete's vertical jump height showed high between-trial reliability but poor concurrent validity when compared to a force plate (i.e., the criterion device) (McMahon et al., 2016). Therefore, such devices may be used reliably to monitor changes in an athlete's vertical jump height over time, but the actual jump height values obtained from the systems are likely to be erroneous, and, therefore, will need to be corrected (i.e., brought in line with force plate jump height values) via published equations (McMahon et al., 2016). Ideally, even modern portable force plates, which are increasingly likely to be used by strength and conditioning coaches (Weldon et al., 2021), should be assessed for agreement with industry gold standard force plates. This has been done for some of the common portable force systems to date via researchers' own algorithms (Lake et al., 2018; Badby et al., 2022), but it should be noted that different commercial force plate software should not be used interchangeably due to poor agreement for many vertical jump variables, even when applied to the same force plate data (Merrigan et al., 2022). For example, there was a 121% difference in countermovement jump propulsive net impulse, which directly influences vertical jump height (Kirby et al., 2011; McBride et al., 2010), between two of the current commercial force plate software leaders (Merrigan et al., 2022).

In the absence of peer-reviewed concurrent validity studies, strength and conditioning coaches may wish to quantify the agreement between the test device they are using and a criterion test device if they are able to collect the required data with their athletes. As concurrent validity is concerned with ascertaining the amount of agreement between two different test devices that purportedly measure the same thing

(Adams et al., 2014), appropriate statistical tests must be applied. A test of mean difference (e.g., a paired t-test) or a correlation test (e.g., Pearson) between the two test devices is insufficient, despite their common application in published concurrent validity studies (Ranganathan et al., 2017). Instead, ordinary least products regression analysis is recommended, as this will inform us as to whether there is any fixed or proportional bias between two methods. Specifically, fixed bias is present if the 95% CIs of the intercept does not include 0. Proportional bias is present if 95% CIs of the slope does not include 1. Fixed bias means that one method produces higher or lower values than those from the other by a constant amount (e.g., always a 2 cm higher difference). Alternatively, proportional bias means that one method produces higher or lower values than the other by an amount that is proportional to the level of the measured variable (Ludbrook, 1997). Good agreement between test devices occurs when there is neither fixed on proportional bias present. The reader is referred to Ludbrook (2010) for more information on ordinary least product regression analyses.

Part 3: Test Administration

To achieve accurate test results, testing needs to be completed in a safe, correct, and organized manner that achieves the goals of the strength and conditioning coach and/or team management. When selecting the specific tests the athletes will complete, the strength and conditioning coach needs to ensure proper health and safety for each athlete. In addition, the coach needs to be properly trained on performance of each test in order to be administered accurately, and the athlete needs to be properly instructed on how to prepare for the upcoming testing session.

Health and Safety Considerations

Prior to testing an athlete, the athlete should be medically cleared and/or a full health screening should be conducted to determine if medical clearance is necessary (see Chapter 1). During each test, the coach needs to be aware of any physical signs and symptoms of any medical issues before, during, or after exertion. Medical referral may be necessary for an athlete that has any of the following symptoms:

- Chest pressure, pain, or discomfort
- Light-headedness, dizziness, blurred vision, or syncope
- Confusion or headache
- Irregular heart rate – too fast or slow
- Bone or joint pain
- Shortness of breath
- Weakness either not commensurate with the level of exertion or unresponsive to rest (McGuigan, 2016).

Selection of Training of Testers

A sporting team may conduct testing on the entire team at the same time and may require additional assistance in testing. These additional testers should be well trained and have a thorough understanding of all tests being conducted. The head strength coach should make sure that all testers perform the testing protocol and score the test the same. It is very important that all testers have sufficient practice to obtain scores that closely correlate with other testers. All testers should explain the tests in a standardized manner and give the same verbal encouragement to make sure that athletes receive similar opportunities to perform the test.

Recording Forms

All tests that are being conducted for a specific testing session should have the proper forms necessary for that day's testing. These test forms can be created by the team or may be downloaded from different books or manuals. Additional information should be documented on the form as well including environmental conditions (room temperature, humidity, time of day), and how the testing was set up, i.e., pin height for barbell in a squat rack or seat height on a machine.

Sequence of Tests

Proper order of tests will ensure test reliability. The central principle of testing sequence should be that one test should not affect the performance of another test. This will allow for optimal performance during each test. When testing consideration of recovery timing is very important as different tests may affect the different energy systems. An example would be a test that affects the phosphagen system (ATP-PC system) would need between 3 and 5 minutes of recovery (Bogdanis et al., 1995).

The proper sequence of tests should be as follows:

1   Non-fatiguing tests – e.g., height, body mass, flexibility, body composition
2   Agility tests – e.g., T-test, pro agility test
3   Maximal power and strength tests – e.g., 1-RM
4   Sprint tests – e.g., 40 m sprint test
5   Muscular endurance – e.g., push-up, curl-up tests
6   Fatiguing anaerobic capacity tests – e.g., Wingate test
7   Aerobic capacity tests – e.g., VO_{2max}, Yo-Yo intermittent test

Preparing Athletes for Testing

Selecting the testing date should include the time of day and announcing to the athlete when to arrive at the facility is important. Prior to the test date, the strength and conditioning coach may consider having the athletes come to the lab facility and allow them to practise performing the tests prior to the main testing day. This will allow the athletes to familiarize themselves with the testing protocol to make sure they know what will be expected from them. Instructions should be given to the athlete prior to testing which include the purpose of testing, how to perform the tests, when to arrive, what to eat prior to testing, and what to wear. The instructions need to be clear and concise to allow the athlete to give their best effort. Prior to testing, a proper warm-up should be given. The warm-up should incorporate a general warm-up and finish with a specific warm-up. The warm-up should include movements that are similar to the testing protocol to follow. Before each test, consider including a few repetitions as a warm-up.

Upon conclusion of testing, a cool-down should be performed after tests that increases heart rate and at the end of the testing battery. The cool-down should include active recovery that incorporates low-intensity movements to enhance the recovery process.

Summary

Strength and conditioning coaches who assess the physical characteristics of their athletes should have an appreciation of the reliability, measurement error, and validity of the devices and metrics that they use. This will allow them to critically interpret the generated data before utilizing it to inform the construction of their athletes' strength and conditioning programs. Strength and conditioning coaches should also invest time in preparing the administrative aspects of testing their athletes to ensure that all testing conducted is as well organized and safe as possible, to facilitate an efficient and ethical performance testing environment.

References

Adams, H., Cervantes, P., Jang, J. & Dixon, D. 2014. Chapter 25 – Standardized assessment. In: Granpeesheh, D., Tarbox, J., Najdowski, A. C. & Kornack, J. (eds). *Evidence-Based Treatment for Children with Autism*. San Diego, CA: Academic Press.

Badby, A. J., Mundy, P., Comfort, P., Lake, J. & Mcmahon, J. J. 2022. *Agreement Among Countermovement Jump Force-Time Variables Obtained from a Wireless Dual Force Plate System and an Industry Gold Standard System*. Liverpool: International Society of Biomechanics in Sports.

Bogdanis, G. C., Nevil, M. E., Boobis, L. H., Lakomy, H. K. A. & Nevill, A. M. 1995. Recovery power output and muscle metabolites following 30 s of maximal sprint cycling in man. *J Appl Physiol*, 482, 467–80.

Borg, D. N., Bach, A. J. E., O'Brien, J. L. & Sainani, K. L. 2022. Calculating sample size for reliability studies. *PM R*, 14, 1018–25.

Claudino, J. G., Cronin, J., Mezêncio, B., Mcmaster, D. T., Mcguigan, M., Tricoli, V., Amadio, A. C. & Serrão, J. C. 2017. The countermovement jump to monitor neuromuscular status: A meta-analysis. *J Sci Med Sport*, 20, 397–402.

Kennedy, R. A. & Drake, D. 2021. Improving the signal-to-noise ratio when monitoring countermovement jump performance. *J Strength Cond Res*, 35, 85–90.

Kirby, T. J., McBride, J. M., Haines, T. L., & Dayne, A. M. (2011). Relative net vertical impulse determines jumping performance. *J Appl Biomech*. 27(3), 207–14.

Koo, T. K. & Li, M. Y. 2016. A guideline of selecting and reporting intraclass correlation coefficients for reliability research. *J Chiropr Med*, 15, 155–63.

Lake, J., Mundy, P., Comfort, P., Mcmahon, J. J., Suchomel, T. J. & Carden, P. 2018. Concurrent validity of a portable force plate using vertical jump force-time characteristics. *J Appl Biomech*, 34, 410–3.

Ludbrook, J. 1997. Comparing methods of measurements. *Clin Exp Pharmacol Physiol*, 24, 193–203.

Ludbrook, J. 2010. Linear regression analysis for comparing two measures or methods of measurement: But which regression? *Clin Exp Pharmacol Physiol*, 37, 692–9.

McBride, J. M., Kirby, T. J., Haines, T. L. & Skinner, J. (2010) Relationship between relative net vertical impulse and jump height in jump squats performed to various squat depths and with various loads. *Int J Sports Physiol Perform*, 5(4), 484–96.

Mcguigan, M. 2016. Principles. Of test selection and administration. In G. Haff & N. T. Triplett (eds), *Essentials of Strength and Conditioning*, 4th ed. Champaign, IL: Human Kinetics. 249–58.

McMahon, J. J., Jones, P. A. & Comfort, P. 2016. A correction equation for jump height measured using the just jump system. *Int J Sports Physiol Perform*, 11, 555–7.

McMahon, J. J., Lake, J. P. & Comfort, P. 2018. Reliability of and relationship between flight time to contraction time ratio and reactive strength index modified. *Sports*, 6, 81.

Merrigan, J. J., Stone, J. D., Galster, S. M. & Hagen, J. A. 2022. Analyzing force-time curves: Comparison of commercially available automated software and custom MATLAB analyses. *J Strength Cond Res*, 36, 2387–402.

Ranganathan, P., Pramesh, C. S. & Aggarwal, R. 2017. Common pitfalls in statistical analysis: Measures of agreement. *Perspect Clin Res*, 8, 187–91.

Shrout, P. E. & Fleiss, J. L. 1979. Intraclass correlations: Uses in assessing rater reliability. *Psychol Bull*, 86, 420–8.

Swinton, P. A., Hemingway, B. S., Saunders, B., Gualano, B. & Dolan, E. 2018. A statistical framework to interpret individual response to intervention: Paving the way for personalized nutrition and exercise prescription. *Front Nutr*, 5, 41.

Weldon, A., Duncan, M. J., Turner, A., Sampaio, J., Noon, M., Wong, D. & Lai, V. W. 2021. Contemporary practices of strength and conditioning coaches in professional soccer. *Biol Sport*, 38, 377–90.

5   Body Composition

Joshua Miller

Part 1: Introduction

Body composition is a key component of an individual's health and physical fitness profile. Athletes today come in all different shapes and sizes and understanding what physical appearance is necessary to compete in the sport of their choice. Appropriate anthropometrics and body composition is necessary for achievement in their sport. Some endurance and power sports are weight dependent, and those athletes that are leaner, i.e., endurance athletes may benefit from a lower percentage of body fat. This benefit of lower percentage body fat may be demonstrated in reduced oxygen consumption during higher intensity exercise when compared to greater weight athletes. However, if percentage body fat is too low in female endurance runners, this may increase the risk of female athlete triad (FAT) or relative energy deficiency in sport (RED-S) (Folscher et al., 2015; Logue et al., 2020). The FAT is a syndrome that involves and interplays between low energy availability, menstrual dysfunction, and altered bone mineral density (Deimel and Dunlan, 2012). RED-S has been demonstrated to occur in male cyclists (Keay et al., 2019) and endurance athletes (Heikura et al., 2018a; Heikura et al., 2018b). Obesity is a serious health problem that affects more than one-third of the population (Williams et al., 2015). However, in certain sports, athletes may have a greater amount of body fat for success in the position. An example would be an offensive lineman in American football. In addition, too little body fatness, seen in individuals in weight-dependent sports or endurance sports, may lead to physiological dysfunction.

It is necessary to understand the underlying theoretical models when assessing body composition. The body is made up of water, protein, minerals, and fat. Certain methods divide the body into two compartments: fat (adipose tissue) mass and fat-free (everything else) mass (Siri 1961; Brozek et al., 1963). Certain assumptions are made when using the two-component model (Gibson, Wagner and Heyward):

1   The density of fat is 0.901 g·cc^{-1}.
2   The density of fat-free mass is 1.100 g·cc^{-1}.
3   The densities of fat and fat-free components are the same for all individuals.
4   The densities of the fat-free mass are constant within an individual, and their proportional contribution to the lean component remains constant.
5   The individual being measured differs from the reference body only in the amount of fat. The fat-free mass of the reference body is assumed to be 73.8% water, 19.4% protein, and 6.8% mineral (Mitchell et al., 1945).

DOI: 10.4324/9781003186762-5

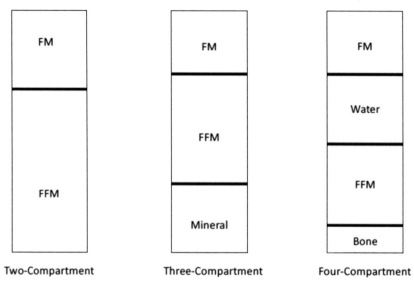

Two-Compartment   Three-Compartment   Four-Compartment

FM = Fat mass; FFM = Fat-Free Mass

Figure 5.1 Two-, three-, and four-compartment body composition models.

The three-compartment model will allow for a direct measurement of bone mineral content and/or total body water. Depending upon available testing equipment utilizing a two-compartment model and measuring a third component will increase the significance of the estimation of percent body fat. The use of DEXA in the exercise physiology laboratory and sporting teams has allowed for a four-compartment mode that controls for biological variability in both total body water (TBW) and bone mineral content. Withers et al. (1999) reported that a multi-compartment technique for body composition can be time-consuming and expensive but is a widely recognized reference method for body composition assessment (see Figure 5.1).

When selecting the body composition technique that will be used to estimate body fat percentage, the tester needs to understand possible error rates and reasons for the error. The ranges can be between 1% and 10% depending upon the technique selected. Traditionally, the gold standard test was hydrostatic weighing and all other techniques have been compared to hydrostatic weighing. Today, the gold standard measurements include densitometry (hydrostatic weighing and air displacement plethysmography [ADP]) and dual-energy X-ray absorptiometry (DEXA) to obtain estimates of body composition. For densitometric methods, total body density (D_b) is estimated from the ratio of body mass (BM) to body volume (BV) ($D_b = BM/BV$). BV can be measured either from hydrodensitometry and ADP.

Proper Clothing Attire for Measurements

When performing any type of body composition measurement, proper clothing should be worn to make measurements as quick and efficient as possible. This means wearing clothing must be of minimal thickness and follow the natural shape of the body to allow access to areas of the skin for skinfolds and other measures. In contrast during tests of hydrodensitometry and/or ADP, spandex shorts for males and spandex shorts and a sports bra for females should be worn to reduce risk of error.

Laboratory Testing

Densitometry

Hydrostatic weighing or underwater weighing (UWW) and ADP (Bod Pod®) are effective, consistent, and widely used laboratory methods for assessing D_b. Densitometry provides an estimate of BV based upon the water and/or air that is displaced by the body's volume. This is based upon Archimedes' principle, which states the weight of a body of water is directly proportional to the volume of water displaced by the body's volume. To calculate Db, BM is divided BV. The total D_b is made up of the amounts of muscle, bone, water, and fat in the body.

Underwater Weighing

To determine BV, the individual is submerged in an UWW tank or pool and the BM of the individual is measured underwater. When measuring the underwater weight, the individual can either be seated in a chair that is attached to scale (see Figure 5.2a) or a platform attached to load cells (see Figure 5.2b). The weight loss from the individual being under water is directly proportional to the volume of water displaced by the body's volume; the BV is equal to BM minus the underwater weight. Some individuals will need additional weight to keep them underwater and this mass is termed the tare weight (TW) and must be subtracted from the underwater weight. Additionally, the BV must be corrected for the volume of air that is remaining in the lungs after a maximal exhalation (this is residual volume (RV)), as well as the gas that is trapped in the gastrointestinal tract (GT). The air in the GT is assumed to be 100 ml.

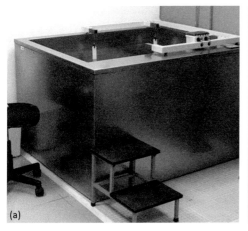
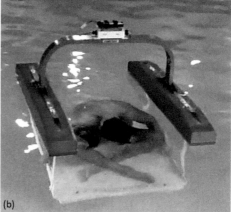

Figure 5.2 (a) and (b) Example of an underwater weighing tank, and individual being submerged. (Photos courtesy of Jeff Tesch, ExerTech.)

RV can be measured directly via a nitrogen washout test. The RV is measured in litres and must be converted to kilograms (kg) to correct the underwater weight. 1 L of air weighs approximately 1 kg, so the conversion is easy to do. To correct BV for air remaining, RV and GT (100 ml or 0.1 kg) must be subtracted from the equation. The density of water must be corrected based upon the temperature of the water and this can affect BV. Thus, the equation for BV is:

$$BV = \left((BM - net\ UWW)/density\ of\ water\right) - (RV + GT)$$

If unable to measure RV via a nitrogen washout test. Several regression models have been created to estimate RV. Calculation of RV can be made by using the RV equations in Table 5.1.

To calculate D_b, divide BM by BV: $D_b = BM - BV$. Once D_b is calculated, it can be converted to percent body fat (%BF) by using the appropriate population-specific conversion formula (see Table 5.2).

Underwater Weighing

Guidelines for Underwater Weighing

Pre-test Guidelines

*   Do not eat or engage in strenuous exercise at least 4 hours prior to testing.
*   Avoid ingesting any gas-producing foods or beverages for at least 12 hours prior to testing.
*   Bring proper attire for the test (i.e., swimsuit).

Testing Procedure Guidelines

*   Prior to testing, make sure the scale is properly calibrated to manufacturer specifications.
*   Encourage the individual to use the restroom to empty their bladder and change into a swimsuit.
*   Measure the individual's BM (dry) to the nearest 0.01 kg.

Table 5.1 Regression equations to estimate residual volume.

	Age (years)	Gender	Equation	Reference
White	15–91	Female	0.0197 (H) + 0.0201 (A) – 2.421	Crapo et al. (1982)
White	15–91	Male	0.0216 (H) + 0.0207 (A) – 2.840	Crapo et al. (1982)
African American	20–60	Female	0.01542 (H) + 0.0230 (A) + 0.00726 (W) – 0.0225 (A) – 2.205	Petersen and Hodous, (1988)
African American	20–60	Male	0.01542 (H) + 0.0230 (A) + 0.00726 (W) – 0.0421 (A) – 2.032	Petersen and Hodous, (1988)

H = height in centimeters; A = age in years; W = body mass in kilograms.

Table 5.2 Population-specific formulas for converting body density to percent body fat.

	Age (years)	Gender	Equation	FF D_b (g.cc-1)	Reference
American Indian	18–60	Female	$(4.81/Db) - 4.34$	1.108	Hicks (1992)
African American	18–32	Male	$(4.37/D_b) - 3.93$	1.113	Schutte et al. (1984)
	24–79	Female	$(4.85/D_b) - 4.39$	1.106	Ortiz et al. (1992)
Hispanic	20–40	Female	$(4.87/D_b) - 4.41$	1.105	Stolarczyk et al. (1995)
White	17–19	Male	$(4.99/D_b) - 4.55$	1.098	Lohman (1986)
		Female	$(5.05/D_b) - 4.62$	1.005	Lohman (1986)
	20–80	Male	$(4.95/D_b) - 4.50$	1.1	Siri (1961)
		Female	$(5.01/D_b) - 4.57$	1.098	Lohman (1986)
			$(4.57/D_b) - 4.142$	1.099	Brozek et al. (1963)
		Athletes			
Endurance	21 ± 2	Male	$(5.03/D_b) - 4.59$	1.097	Gibson et al. (2019)
	21 ± 4	Female	$(4.95/D_b) - 4.50$	1.1	Siri 1961
Resistance	24 ± 4	Male	$(5.21/D_b) - 4.78$	1.089	Gibson et al. (2019)
	35 ± 6	Female	$(4.97/D_b) - 4.52$	1.099	Gibson et al. (2019)

- Check and record the water temperature of the tank or pool before the test. The temperature should range between 34 and 36°C (see Table 5.3 to determine the density of water at the temperature recorded.
- Ask the individual to shower prior to entering the water. Once entering the water, ask them to be as calm as possible so the water does not become rough which could affect the test. Ask the individual to submerge themselves in the water and rub down their body and hair to remove any air bubbles that are trapped on their skin or swimsuit.
- Have the individual sit on chair or kneel on the platform. Additional weight may need to be given to completely submerge the individual underwater when they perform the test.

Table 5.3 Density of water at various temperatures.

Water Temperature	Density Value
25°C	0.99707
26°C	0.99681
27°C	0.99654
28°C	0.99626
29°C	0.99597
30°C	0.99567
31°C	0.99537
32°C	0.99505
33°C	0.99471
34°C	0.99438
35°C	0.99404
36°C	0.99369
37°C	0.99333

- Ask them to take a few normal breaths and then exhale maximally while slowly bending forward to submerge the body. Make sure that their head is completely submerged as well. If any part of their body is not submerged tap them gently to try to submerge it further. Once they have reached RV, they should remain as still as possible for a count of 5 for an accurate measurement to be made.
- Record the highest measurement during the trail and signal them that the trail is complete.
- Administer the test for a maximum of ten trials. Many individuals will achieve consistent and maximal trials within 4–5 trials. Average the three highest trials.
- Prior to exiting the take, ask the individual to place the weight on the chair or platform for measurement of the TW.
- Determine the true UWW by subtracting the TW from the gross UWW. This will be the net UWW.

Tips for Minimizing Error During Hydrostatic Weighing
- Make sure all pre-test guidelines have been met.
- Make sure calibration for all equipment is completed properly.
- Precisely measure BV to ± 50 g, UWW to ± 100 g, and RV to ± 100 ml.
- Practise maximally exhaling all air to RV and remaining as still as possible.
- As the individual submerges, try to steady the scale, but when the measurement is taken, do not touch the scale.
- When calculating Db, carry the value to at least 5 decimal places to reduce error.
- Select the proper population-specific conversion formula (see Table 5.1).

Data Analysis and Interpretation

Once the proper population-specific conversion formula has been used to determine percentage body fat, calculation of fat-free mass and fat mass can be made.

- Fat mass = Body mass × percent body fat (in decimal)
- Fat-free mass = Body mass – fat mass

Additionally, percentage body fat can be utilized to determine the proper body fat percentage category of body fat (see Table 5.4). Table 5.5 illustrates body composition characteristics of different types of sporting athletes.

Air Displacement Plethysmography (ADP)

ADP is a second method to determine BV and Db. This technique uses air displacement to estimate volume instead of water. This technique is relatively quick (~7–10 minutes) and requires very little compliance by the individual, and minimal technician skill, it is considered an alternative to hydrostatic weighing. The Bod Pod is a device that utilizes ADP to estimate BV. The Bod Pod is an egg-shaped fiberglass chamber that uses air displacement and pressure-volume (P-V) relationships to estimate BV (see Figure 5.3).

The Bod Pod is a device that uses a dual-chamber system to estimate BV (Figure 5.4). The individual will sit in the front chamber and the chamber behind the individual

Table 5.4 Body fat percentage categories for males and females.

Age	Very Lean (%)	Lean (%)	Average (%)	Over Fat (%)	Obese (%)
			Males		
20–29	4–7	8–12	13–17	18–23	>23
30–39	7–11	12–16	17–20	21–25	>25
40–49	9–13	14–18	19–22	23–26	>26
50–59	11–15	16–20	21–23	24–28	>28
60–69	12–17	18–21	22–24	25–29	>29
70–79	14–16	17–21	22–24	25–29	>29
			Females		
20–29	11–15	16–18	19–22	23–28	>28
30–39	11–16	17–19	20–23	24–30	>30
40–49	12–17	18–21	22–25	26–32	>32
50–59	13–19	20–24	25–28	29–34	>34
60–69	14–20	21–25	26–29	30–35	>35
70–79	11–18	19–24	25–28	29–25	>35

is a reference chamber. Between the chambers is a large diaphragm that oscillates during the test. The P-V relationship is used to calculate the volume for the front chamber when it is empty and when the individual sits in the chair. BV is calculated as the difference in the volume in the chamber with and without the individual inside of the device.

Table 5.5 Body composition characteristics of athletes.

Sport	Gender	% Body Fat	Technique	Reference
Baseball – MLB	M	14.9 + 6.4	SKF	Coleman and Lasky (1992)
Basketball – NBA	M	7.2 + 1.9	SKF	Gonzalez et al. (2013)
Road Cyclist – Professional	M	10.1 + 1.2	BIA	Marra et al. (2016)
Distance Running – DI	F	18.3 + 2.7	DEXA	Fornetti et al. (1999)
Field Hockey – DI	F	20.9 + 4.1	DEXA	Fornetti et al. (1999)
Football – DI	M	17.0 + 6.6	UWW	Collins et al. (1999)
Football – DII	M	11.9 + 3.4	SKF	Mayhew et al. (1989)
Gymnastics	F	19.1 + 2.2	DEXA	Fornetti et al. (1999)
Hockey – Collegiate	M	16.1 + 3.9	DEXA	Chiarlitti et al. (2017)
Rowing – DI	F	22.2 + 7.3	UWW	Vescovi et al. (2002)
Soccer – DI	F	21.8 + 2.7	DEXA	Fornetti et al. (1999)
Soccer – Seniors	M	11.6 + 3.7	BIA	Spehnjak et al. (2021)
Softball – DI	F	21.7 + 5.7	UWW	Vescovi et al. (2002)
Swimming – DI	M	15.1 + 3.8	UWW	Prior et al. (2001)
Swimming – DI	F	23.5 + 5.8	UWW	Prior et al. (2001)
Track and Field – DI	F	15.7 + 4.5	UWW	Vescovi et al. (2002)
Volleyball – DI	F	19.1 + 2.7	SKF	Fry et al. (1991)
Weightlifting – US national	M	20.4 + 1.9	SKF	Fry et al. (1991)
Wrestling – DI	M	7.3 + 0.7	SKF	Kraemer et al. (1991)

SKF = skinfold; BIA = bioelectric impedance; UWW = underwater weighing; DEXA = dual energy X-ray absorptiometry.

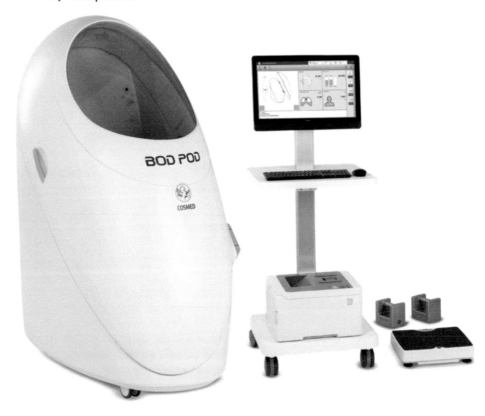

Figure 5.3 Bod Pod GS-X. (Courtesy of COSMED, USA. From https://www.cosmed.com/
hires/Bodpod_GS-X_Brochure_A3_4pages_C05140-02-93_EN_print.pdf.)

The underlying principle for ADP is the relationship between pressure and volume. At a constant temperature (isothermal condition), volume (V), and pressure (P) are inversely related. According to Boyle's law,

$$P_1/P_2 = V_2/V_1$$

where P_1 and V_1 represent one paired condition of P and V, and P_2 and V_2 represent another paired condition.

- P_1 and V_1 represent when the Bod Pod is empty, and
- P_2 and V_2 represent when an individual is in the Bod Pod.

An assumption made is that the Bod Pod controls the isothermal effects of clothing, hair, thoracic gas volume (TGV), and body surface area (BSA) while the individual is seated in the chamber. When undergoing a test, individuals wear minimal clothing (i.e., swimsuit), and a swim cap to compress the hair. BSA is calculated from the height and BM of the individual that is inputted into the computer. TGV is calculated from the functional residual capacity (FRC) at mid-exhalation. TGV can be estimated or measured directly during the test to account for isothermal conditions in

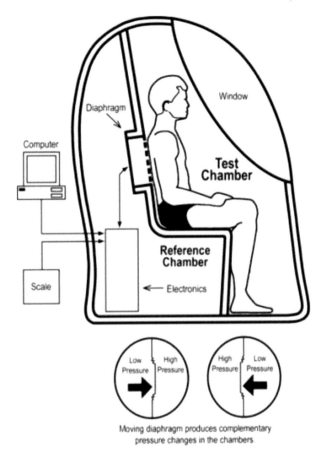

Figure 5.4 Bod Pod device schematic, including visualization of diaphragm perturbations utilized to determine body volume of the participant in the measurement chamber. (Courtesy of COSMED, USA. Schematic from http://www.cosmed.com/hires/marketing_literature/product_news/Product_News_Air_Displacement_EN_print.pdf.)

the lungs. Several studies have demonstrated that the estimation of TGV can be used instead of measuring it during the test (McCrory et al., 1998; Demerath et al., 2002; Henricksson et al., 2013; Miller 2016).

Air Displacement Plethysmography

Guidelines for ADP

Pre-test Guidelines

- Do not eat or engage in strenuous exercise at least 4 hours prior to testing.
- Avoid ingesting any gas-producing foods or beverages for at least 12 hours prior to testing.
- Have the individual empty their bladder and bowel.
- Bring proper attire for the test (i.e., swimsuit).

- Follow manufacturer guidelines for calibration.

  - Be careful when handling the calibration cylinder to make sure no dents or damage are made as this can affect calibration of the Bod Pod®.

Testing Procedure Guidelines

- Instruct the individual to change into dry, form-fitting swimwear. Females should wear either a one-piece bathing suit or sports bra and compression shorts. Males should wear either a swimsuit (i.e., speedo) or compression shorts (without padding).
- Prior to testing, measure the individual's height to the nearest centimeter on a stadiometer.
- Follow guidelines for inputting the individual's information (name, date of birth, ethnicity [either general population or African American only choices], and height).
- Begin two-point calibration of the Bod Pod and measure BM using the scale that is attached to the device.
- Once instructed by the device, ask the individual to sit inside of the front chamber while wearing the swim cap. Make sure that no additional clothing is worn besides the swimsuit and the swim cap.

  - Remind them that the door will be magnetically sealed and airtight.
  - Ask them to breathe normal.
  - Once the door is closed, it will take approximately 30 seconds to complete the first test.

- Follow the prompts on the computer screen, open the door fully, and then close the door for the second measurement.

  - If the two tests are off by 150 ml, repeat the test for a third time.

- Ask the individual to exit the Bod Pod.

Tips for Minimizing Error During ADP

- Make sure all pre-test guidelines have been met.
- Make sure calibration for all equipment is completed properly.
- Make sure the individual is wearing the proper clothing and swim cap during the test.
- Avoid any movement while the test is ongoing.

Data Analysis and Interpretation

Figure 5.5 is the printout that the Bod Pod creates when a test is ended. At the beginning of the test, inputting the correct gender and ethnicity will select the proper database for comparison of percent body fat. The population-specific conversion formula will be selected based upon the ethnicity of the individual (general population or African American). However, Brozek, Siri, Schutte (Black only), or Lohman (children or adolescents) equations can be selected based upon the desire of the tester (Lohman, T.G. et al., 1988). Similar results will be determined upon printout from the device (see Figure 5.5).

BOD POD® Body Composition Tracking System Analysis

SUBJECT INFORMATION	
NAME	michael moore
AGE	44
GENDER	Male
HEIGHT	71.0 in
ID_1	
ID_2	
ETHNICITY	General Population
OPERATOR	wfc
TEST DATE	July 22, 2010
TEST NUMBER	926

BODY COMPOSITION RESULT		
% FAT	44.9	%
% FAT FREE MASS	55.1	%
FAT MASS	122.249	lb
FAT FREE MASS	149.939	lb
BODY MASS	272.189	lb
BODY VOLUME	123.441	L
BODY DENSITY	1.0002	kg/L
THORACIC GAS VOLUME	4.221	L

OPERATOR COMMENTS

TEST PROFILE	
DENSITY MODEL	Siri
THORACIC GAS VOLUME MODEL	Predicted

Body Fat: A certain amount of fat is absolutely necessary for good health. Fat plays an important role in protecting internal organs, providing energy, and regulating hormones. The minimal amount of "essential fat" is approximately 3-5% for men, and 12-15% for women. If too much fat accumulates over time, health may be compromised (see table below).

Fat Free Mass: Fat free mass is everything except fat. It includes muscle, water, bone, and internal organs. Muscle is the "metabolic engine" of the body that burns calories (fat) and plays an important role in maintaining strength and energy. Healthy levels of fat-free mass contribute to physical fitness and may prevent conditions such as osteoporosis.

LMI Body Fat Rating Table*

*Applies to adults ages 18 and older. Based on information from the American College of Sports Medicine, the American Council on Exercise, Exercise Physiology (4th Ed.) by McArdle, Katch, and Katch, and various scientific and epidemiological studies.

	BODY FAT RATING	MALE	EXPLANATION
X	Risky (high body fat)	> 30%	Ask your health care professional about how to safely modify your body composition.
	Excess Fat	20 - 30%	Indicates an excess accumulation of fat over time.
	Moderately Lean	12 - 20%	Fat level is generally acceptable for good health.
	Lean	8 - 12%	Lower body fat levels than many people. This range is generally excellent for health and longevity.
	Ultra Lean	5 - 8%	Fat levels often found in elite athletes.
	Risky (low body fat)	< 5%	Ask your health care professional about how to safely modify your body composition.

ENERGY EXPENDITURE RESULTS

Est. Resting Metabolic Rate (RMR) kcal/day	*Est. Total Energy Expenditure (TEE) kcal/day	Daily Activity Level
1979 (See RMR Info Sheet for additional info)	2533	Sedentary
	2988	Low Active
	3443	Active
	4116	Very Active
	*Est. TEE = Est. RMR x Daily Activity Level	

Applies to adults ages 18 and older. Based on information from the Institute of Medicine (2002), Dietary Reference Intakes For Energy, Carbohydrate, Fiber, Fat, Fatty Acids, Cholesterol, Protein, And Amino Acids, Part I, pp93-206. Washington, D.C., National Academy of Sciences.

 Life Measurement, Inc. • 1-800-4 BOD POD • www.lifemeasurement.com

Figure 5.5 Example of a printout from the Bod Pod. (Courtesy of the UIC Human Performance Laboratory.)

Dual-Energy X-Ray Absorptiometry

DEXA/DXA is becoming one of the most widely used devices to estimate body composition (Figure 5.6). In addition, it is also considered a reference method for body composition in research and clinical settings. This technique divides the body into three compartments – bone mineral, fat (adipose and visceral adipose tissue (VAT)), and fat-free mass. The test can compare whole-body and regional (trunk and appendicular) levels of the different compartments. DEXA is safe and time-efficient when comparing to UWW because it requires some compliance by the individual but will require the tester to be well trained. A whole-body scan can be completed within 5–7 minutes depending upon the type of DEXA (Bazzocchi et al., 2016).

The technology of the DEXA is the reduction of X-rays with high and low photon energies measurable and dependent upon the thickness, density, and chemical composition of the underlying tissues (Gibson et al. 2019). This reduction of X-ray energies is called attenuation. Tissues have different attenuations based upon the differences of density and chemical composition of the tissues. An assumption of these X-ray ratios for the high and low energies is thought to be constant for all individuals (Pietrobelli et al., 1996). The amount of radiation that is given off by the device is

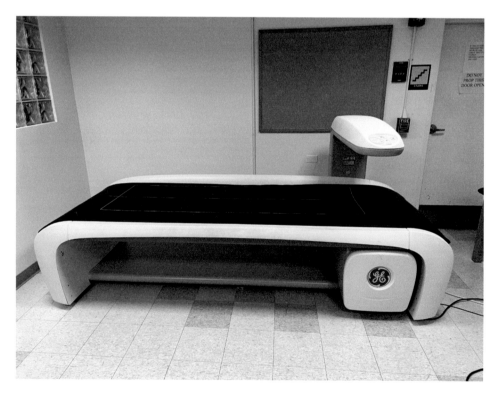

Figure 5.6 Dual-energy X-ray absorptiometry (DEXA) device, GE lunar prodigy series. (Photo taken at the University of Illinois Chicago Integrative Physiology Laboratory, Chicago, IL.)

very minimal. An individual will receive more radiation while flying in a plane than completing the test.

There are several different types of DEXA devices in the market (GE, Hologic, and Norland) and each has its own proprietary software that makes it difficult to assess the validity of the devices. This leads to issues upon standardization of the test. Lohman et al. (2000) reviewed studies using DEXA and concluded DEXA estimates body fat percentage within 1–3% of multi-compartment methods. Several studies have concluded that DEXA is a better predictor than UWW (Friedl et al., 1992; Prior et al., 1997; Wagner and Heyward, 2001). However, there have been studies that reported that DEXA is not as accurate as UWW (Bergsma-Kadijk et al., 1996; Millard-Stafford et al., 2001).

Guidelines for DEXA/DXA

Pre-test Guidelines

- Calibrate device to manufacturer standards using the calibration block provided by manufacturer.
- Have the individual void his bladder and bowel and remove all jewelry.
- Measure the individual's height and BM while wearing as minimal clothing as possible. Make sure there is no metal in any undergarments.

Testing Procedure Guidelines

- Instruct the individual to lie suping (on his back) on the scanner bed.
- Some scanners will automatically make adjustment based upon body thickness.
- Make sure the individual holds his arms in a neutral position next to his body during the scan.
- Consider using a Velcro strap on his knees to make sure of no movement.
- Have the individual lie as still as possible as he is being scanned.

Data Analysis and Interpretation

DEXA produces a printout that illustrates percent fat based upon entire body, body segments (i.e., arms, legs, and trunk), and right and left sides of the body (Figure 5.7). Additionally, bone density is determined based upon the scan of the whole body.

Field Testing

In field testing, techniques can be utilized that do not require expensive equipment but still need proper training on the equipment. The coach has several different types of equipment to select from including skinfolds, bioelectrical impedance analysis (BIA), ultrasound, and other types of prediction equations. As with the laboratory tests, the coach needs to understand the basic assumptions and principles as well as sources of error for each method. Each technique has established standardized testing protocols that need to be followed and should be practised reducing the potential for error. All field tests have been validated to the reference tests to make sure the test can reproduce similar results.

UIC
Kinesiology and Nutrition,
Phone: (___) ___-___

Patient:	001, 001			Referring Physician: (not specified)	
Birth Date:	02/12/1989	Age:	30.6 years	Patient ID:	001
Height:	67.0 in.	Weight:	149.8 lbs.	Measured:	09/24/2019 1:16:30 PM (17 [SP 1])
Sex:	Male	Ethnicity:	White	Analyzed:	09/24/2019 1:16:34 PM (17 [SP 1])

Total Body Tissue Quantitation

Composition (Enhanced Analysis)

Region	Tissue (%Fat)	Centile	Total Mass (kg)	Fat (g)	Lean (g)	BMC (g)
Arms	11.4	-	9.2	995	7,725	492
Legs	13.9	-	20.9	2,755	17,066	1,036
Trunk	16.0	-	33.7	5,262	27,656	810
Android	16.4	-	4.7	764	3,883	53
Gynoid	15.5	-	10.3	1,558	8,461	316
Total	15.1	25	68.4	9,866	55,672	2,888

Total Body: Total

Tissue (%Fat)

Total Body: Total (Total Mass)

%Change vs Previous

USA (Lunar)

USA (Combined NHANES/Lunar) Trend: Total (Enhanced Analysis)

Measured Date	Age (years)	Tissue (%Fat)	Centile	Total Mass (kg)	Tissue (g)	Fat (g)	Lean (g)	BMC (g)	Fat Free (g)
09/24/2019	30.6	15.1	25	68.4	65,537	9,866	55,672	2,888	58,559

USA (Combined NHANES/Lunar) Trend: Fat Distribution (Enhanced Analysis)

Measured Date	Age (years)	Android (%Fat)	Gynoid (%Fat)	A/G Ratio	Total (%Fat)
09/24/2019	30.6	16.4	15.5	1.06	15.1

World Health Organization BMI Classification

BMI = 23.5 (kg/m^2)

13	18.5	25	30	35
Underweight	Normal	Overweight	Obese	

| 83 | 118 | 160 | 192 | 223 |

Weight (lbs.) for height = 67.0 in.

Color Mapping (%Fat)
25%   60%

Image not for diagnosis

COMMENTS:

Statistically 68% of repeat scans fall within 1SD (± 0.4 % Fat, ±150 g Tissue Mass, ±280 g Fat Mass, ±310 g Lean Mass for Total Body Total). USA (Lunar) Total Body Composition, Male Reference Population (v1.13); Composition Matched for Age, Sex
Date created: 08/29/2022 3:35:21 PM 17 [SP 1] Filename: 88icyp45y.meb; Total Body: 100.0.19:153.85:15.6 0.00:-1.00 2.40a3.04 11.8:%Fat=15.1%, 0.00:0.00 0.00:0.00, Scan Mode Standard 3.0 µGy

GE Healthcare   Page: 1 of 1   Lunar iDXA   ME+210166

Figure 5.7 Example of a printout-form DEXA device for body composition. (Courtesy of the UIC Human Performance Laboratory.)

Anthropometry

Anthropometry refers to the measurement of the human body. It is one of the most common techniques used to describe the individual in human performance. Height and BM not only serve to describe the individual but also contributes to the overall fitness assessment.

Height and Body Mass

Height and BM are the most common techniques used in the research laboratory and the strength and conditioning facility. When measuring height, the individual will remove his shoes and stands against a wall. On the wall may be an attached tape measure or a device called a stadiometer (see Figure 5.8). While the individual is standing fully erect, an object or measuring device is lowered to the top of the head and the measurement is read. Height should be measured to the nearest 0.5 cm (0.25 in). Calibration can be conducted on each device using a tape measurement to confirm the measurement.

BM is measured using a calibrated electronic or certified balance scale (see Figure 5.9). The individual should be wearing a T-shirt, shorts, and no shoes. Measurement should be taken after the individual voids his bladder, and to ensure the lightest

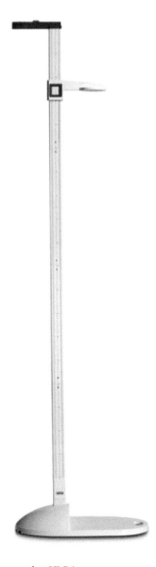

Figure 5.8 Example of a stadiometer by SECA.

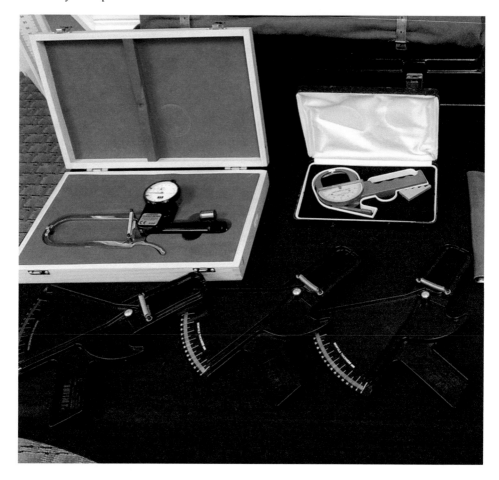

Figure 5.9 Different skinfold callipers for the measurement of skinfolds. (Photos courtesy by Kelley Altom, MS.)

measurement of the day, consider rising in the morning after using the restroom. All measurements should be taken at similar times of the day to ensure consistency. Body mass is reported to the nearest kg (0.1 lb).

Body Mass Index

The body mass index (BMI) is calculated by dividing BM in kilograms (kg) by height in meters squared (m^2). BMI is used in epidemiological studies to stratify individuals into obesity and assess disease risk. One issue associated with BMI is that it does not differentiate based upon FFM and FM. As a result, this is not an appropriate technique used with athletic populations. Table 5.6 classifies the different BMI categories.

Standardized Procedures for Height and Body Mass

These measurements are very easy to measure.

Table 5.6 Body mass index categories.

Category	BMI (kg/m²)
Underweight	< 18.5
Normal	18.5–24.9
Overweight	25.0–29.9
Obese (class I)	30.0–34.9
Obese (class II)	35.0–39.9
Extremely obese (class III)	> 40.0

1 Prior to testing, ensure the individual has emptied his bladder.
2 Remove shoes and measure the individual in a T-shirt, a pair of shorts, and socks only or as minimal clothing as possible.
3 When measuring the individual's height, ensure his heels are against the wall and he is standing as erect as possible.
4 When measuring BM, make sure the individual is standing in the middle of the platform and have him not move while performing the measurement.

Data Analysis and Interpretation

The reader is referred to the National Center for Health Statistics for comparison of height and BM based on age, gender, and ethnicity (In the United States: https://www.cdc.gov/nchs/data/series/sr_03/sr03-046-508.pdf, (Fryar et al., 2021), In the UK: https://digital.nhs.uk/data-and-information/publications/statistical/health-survey-for-england/2019) (Lifestyles Team, NHS Digital, 2020)).

Skinfold Testing

Skinfold testing indirectly measures the thickness of subcutaneous adipose tissue. Skinfold testing can be used to estimate total Db to calculate percentage body fat. Skinfold prediction equations are developed using either a linear (population-specific) or quadratic (generalized) regression models. As we noted earlier, there are several different population-specific formulas for converting Db to percent body fat. There are many different types of equations for estimating Db from skinfolds, circumferences, and bony diameters (Jackson and Pollock, 1985). Table 5.7 lists several different skinfold prediction equations for different populations. Figure 5.9 illustrates the different tools for estimation of body composition from field testing.

Standardized Procedures for Skinfold Measurements

Skinfold measurements take a great amount of time and practice to develop skills to be a skilled tester. There are different standardized protocols that can be selected from to produce reliable and accurate measurements.

1 All skinfold measurements should be taken on the right side of the body unless there is an issue with the specific site being tested.

Table 5.7 Skinfold prediction equations.

Skinfold Sites	Population	Equation	Reference
Σ7SKF	Black or Hispanic women, 18–55 yr	D_b (g·cc⁻¹) = 1.0970 – 0.00046971 × (Σ7SKF) + 0.00000056 × (Σ7SKF)² – 0.00012828 × (age)	Jackson et al. (1980)
Σ7SKF	Black men or male athletes, 18–61 yr	D_b (g·cc⁻¹) = 1.1120 – 0.00043499 × (Σ7SKF) + 0.00000055 × (Σ7SKF)² – 0.00028826 × (age)	Jackson and Pollock (1978)
Σ4SKF	Female athletes, 18–29 yr	D_b (g·cc⁻¹) = 1.096095 – 0.0006952 × (Σ4SKF) + 0.0000011 (Σ4SKF)² – 0.0000714 × (age)	Jackson et al. (1980)
Σ3SKF (female)	White or anorexic women, 18–55 yr	D_b (g·cc⁻¹) = 1.0994921 – 0.0009929 × (Σ3SKF) + 0.0000023 × (Σ3SKF)² – 0.0001392 × (age)	Jackson et al. (1980)
Σ3SKF (male)	White men, 18–61 yr	D_b (g·cc⁻¹) = 1.109380 – 0.0008267 × (Σ3SKF) + 0.0000016 × (Σ3SKF)² – 0.0002574 × (age)	Jackson and Pollock (1978)
Σ3SKF (athlete)	Black or white collegiate male and female athletes, 18–34 yr	% BF = 8.997 + 0.2468 × (Σ3SKF) – 6.343 × (gender) – 1.998 × (race)	Evans et al. (2005)
Σ2SKF (youth)	Black or white boys and girls, 6–17 yr	% BF = 0.735 × (Σ2SKF) + 1.0 % BF = 0.610 × (Σ3SKF) + 5.1	Slaughter et al. (1988)

ΣSKF = sum of skinfolds (mm); Σ7SKF = (chest + abdomen + triceps + thigh + subscapular + suprailliac + midaxillary); S4SKF = (triceps + anterior suprailliac + abdomen + thigh); SSKF (female) = (triceps + suprailliac + thigh); S3SKF (male) = (chest + abdomen + thigh); S3SKF (athlete) = (abdomen + thigh + triceps) (gender − male athletes = 1; female athletes = 0) (race − black athletes = 1; white athletes = 0). (American College of Sports Medicine, 2021)

2 Carefully identify, measure, and mark the skinfold site.
3 Grasp the skinfold firmly between the thumb and index finger of your left hand. Lift the fold 1 cm (0.4 in) above the site to measure.

   a If the individual has very large skinfolds, a larger separation of fingers when grasping the skinfold site may be necessary.

4 Keep the fold elevated while taking the measurement.
5 Place the jaws of the caliper perpendicular to the fold, approximately 1 cm (0.4 in) below the thumb and index finger and halfway between the crest and the base of the fold.

   a Release the jaw of the caliper pressure slowly.

6 Hold the site in the jaws of the calipers for 2–3 seconds before taking the reading.
7 Open the jaws of the caliper to remove it from the site before closing the jaws of the calipers.

Recommendations for Skinfold Testing

• When locating the anatomical landmarks, measuring the distance, and marking the site with a marker be very accurate.

- Read the dial on the caliper to the nearest 0.1 mm (Harpenden) 0.5 mm (Lange), or 1 mm (plastic calipers) (see Figure 5.9).
- A minimum of two measurements at each site is required. If the values are greater than 2 mm, complete a third measurement and average the two measurements that are the closest.
- Rotate the skinfold measurements rather than repeating the same measurement.
- Make sure the individual's skin is dry and free from body lotion.
- Do not conduct testing after exercise because it can cause an error due to extra water within the muscles.
- Practise on more than 50 individuals to become very proficient in technique.
- Seek a mentor who you can compare your results with.

Data Analysis and Interpretation

The population-specific conversion formula will be selected based upon the ethnicity of the individual (see Table 5.4).

Case Study

You are the strength and conditioning coach for a football club. The head coach has asked you to test a player that has been on the injured for the past three months. The coach has asked to estimate his current percentage body fat. You decide to use the seven-site SKF test. Upon completion, you record the following information:

Player: 23-year-old male	% BF SKF = 18.1%
Body mass: 72 kg (158.4 lb)	% BF prior to injury = 13.2%
Height: 165.1 cm (65 in.)	BMI = 26.4 kg/m²
Σ 7SKF: 132 mm	Body Density – 1.07833 g·cc⁻¹

Upon collection of the data and analysis of the SKFs, it was determined that the player has increased his fat mass percentage as well as their normal BM. The athlete will be referred to the team dietician to aide in reduction of BM and percent fat to get back to their pervious BM prior to their injury.

Bioelectrical Impedance Analysis

BIA is a quick, non-invasive test that is used to evaluate body composition in the field. This technique measures a low-level electrical current that is passed through the body, and the impedance, or opposition to the flow of current is measured with an analyzer (see Figure 5.10). TBW can be estimated from the impedance measurement because the electrolytes in the body's water are an excellent conductor of electrical current. When TBW is high, the current flows more easily through the body, due to less resistance. The opposite is demonstrated in individuals with higher levels of adipose tissue, which is due to lower levels of water content in the tissue, the current flows less easily due to more resistance. Fat-free mass can be predicted from TBW estimates (an assumption is the body is made up of ~ 73% water). Individuals with increased FFM and TBW will have less resistance to the current flowing through their bodies than someone with lower FFM. BIA indirectly estimates FFM and TBW based

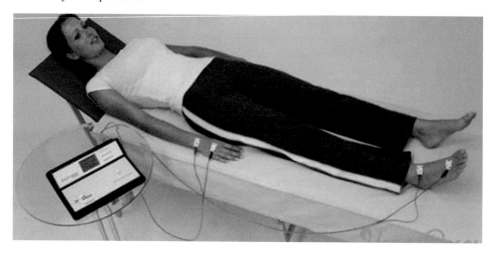

Figure 5.10 Bioelectric impedance analysis using the RJL Systems device.

upon the following assumptions made about the shape of the body and the relationship of impedance to the length and volume of the conductor:

- The human body is shaped like a perfect cylinder with uniform length and cross-sectional area.
- The impedance is directly related to the length of the conductor (height) and inversely related to the cross-sectional area.
- Tissues act as conductors or insulators, and the flow of current through the body will follow the path of least resistance.

There are different types of BIA testing devices on the market currently (see Figure 5.10). These include whole body, upper body (hand-to-hand), and lower body (foot-to-foot). The upper and lower body devices have been made to be used in the home and/or laboratory.

Pre-test Guidelines for BIA Testing

- Avoid eating or drinking within 4 hours of the test.
- No moderate or vigorous exercise within 12 hours of the test.
- Have the individual empty their bladder within 30 minutes of the test.
- Avoid alcohol consumption within 48 hours of the test.
- Do not take any diuretic medication, unless prescribed by a physician, or consume any caffeine prior to the test.
- Consider postponing test during menstrual cycle that the individual may be retaining water.

Standardized Procedures for Whole-Body BIA Testing

1 All measurements will be taken on the right side of the body, while the individual is lying in supine on a non-conductive surface in a room with normal ambient temperature (~25°C/~77°F).

2　Clean the skin where the electrodes will be placed on the hand and foot with an alcohol wipe.

3　Place the proximal electrode on the dorsal surface of the wrist so that the electrode is between the ulna and radius and the second proximal electrode on the dorsal surface of the ankle between the medial and lateral malleoli (see Figure 5.10).

4　Place the distal electrode on the dorsal surface of the hand and foot at the bases of the second and third metacarpophalangeal joints (see Figure 5.10). There should be at least 5 cm (~ 2 in) between the proximal and distal electrodes.

5　Attach the wires to the correct electrodes. Red leads will be attached to the wrist and ankle while the black electrodes will be attached to the hand and foot.

6　The individual's arms and legs should be abducted slightly, ~ 30°–45° angle from the body. Make sure there is no contact between the arms and trunk and the thighs cannot touch either as this can affect the test results.

Data Analysis and Interpretation

Once results are determined from BIA, select the proper population-specific equation to determine FFM (see Table 5.8).

If the individual is lean, use the equations marked < 20% (male) or < 30% (female). If the individual is obese, use the equations marked ≥ 20% (male) or ≥ 30% (female).

Table 5.8 Bioelectric impedance analysis population-specific equations.

Population	% BF Level	Equation	Reference
American Indian, black, Hispanic, or white male, 17–62 yr	< 20% BF	FFM (kg) = $0.00066360 \times (ht^2) - 0.02117 \times (R) + 0.62854 \times (BM) - 0.12380 \times (age) + 9.33285$	Segal et al. (1988)
American Indian, black, Hispanic, or white male, 17–62 yr	> 20% BF	FFM (kg) = $0.00088580 \times (ht^2) - 0.02999 \times (R) + 0.42688 \times (BM) - 0.07002 \times (age) + 14.52435$	Segal et al. (1988)
American Indian, black, Hispanic, or white female, 17–62 yr	< 30% BF	FFM (kg) = $0.000646 \times (ht^2) - 0.014 \times (R) + 0.421 \times (BM) + 10.4$	Segal et al. (1988)
American Indian, black, Hispanic, or white female, 17–62 yr	> 30% BF	FFM (kg) = $0.00091186 \times (ht^2) - 0.01466 \times (R) + 0.299990 \times (BM) - 0.07012 \times (age) + 9.37938$	Segal et al. (1988)
White boys and girls, 8–15 yr	N/A	FFM (kg) = $0.62 \times (ht^2/R) + 0.25 \times (BM) + 0.10 (X_c) + 4.2$	Lohman (1992)
White boys and girls, 10–19 yr	N/A	FFM (kg) = $0.61 \times (ht^2/R) + 0.21 \times (BM) + 1.31$	Houtkooper et al. (1992)
Female athletes, 18–27 yr	N/A	FFM (kg) = $0.282 \times (ht) + 0.415 \times (BM) - 0.37 \times (R) + 0.096 (X_c) - 9.734$	Fornetti et al. (1999)
Male athletes, 19–40 yr	N/A	FFM (kg) = $0.186 \times (ht^2/R) + 0.701 \times (BM) + 1.949$	Oppliger et al. (1991)

%BF = percent body fat; FFM = fat-free mass (kg); ht = height (cm); BM = body mass (kg); R = resistance (Ω); X_c = reactance (Ω); N/A = non-applicable.

If unsure, use both equations and average the values found for both equations to estimate FFM.

Part 2: Practical Examples

Case Study 1: Skinfold Testing

Prior to the football (US soccer) season starting, the head coach has asked you to complete skinfold testing on one of the forwards. During the off-season, she has focused on weight loss and the coach wants to make sure that she has not sacrificed a lot of fat-free muscle mass through dieting.

At the end of the season, the athlete's BM was 69 kg and percent body fat was 24% (16.6 kg FM; 52.4 kg FFM). Data collected are presented in Table 5.9.

Table 5.9 Skinfold site locations.

Site	Direction of Fold	Anatomic Reference	Measurement
Chest	Diagonal	Axilla and nipple	One-half the distance between the anterior axillary line and the nipple (men) or one-third of the distance between the anterior axillary line and the nipple (women).
Triceps	Vertical	Acromion process of scapula and olecranon process of ulna	Posterior midline of the upper arm, halfway between the acromion process and olecranon process.
Subscapular	Diagonal	Inferior angle of scapula	1–2 cm below the inferior angle of the scapula.
Midaxillary	Horizontal	Mid axilla intersects with a horizontal line level with the bottom edge of the xiphoid process	On the midaxillary line at the level of the xiphoid process of the sternum.
Suprailliac	Oblique	Iliac crest	In line with the natural angle of the iliac crest taken in the anterior axillary line immediately superior to the crest.
Abdominal	Horizontal	Umbilicus	2 cm to the right of the umbilicus.
Thigh	Vertical	Inguinal crease and patella	On the anterior midline of the thigh, midway between the proximal border of the patella and the inguinal crease.
Biceps	Vertical	Biceps brachii	On the anterior aspect of the arm over the belly of the biceps, 1 cm above the level of the triceps site.
Calf	Vertical	Maximal calf circumference	On the midline of the medial border of the calf.

Source: Adapted from ACSM GETP 11ed. ISAK.

Gender: F   Body Mass: 65 kg   Age: 22 years

Measurement	Trial 1	Trial 2	Trial 3	Average
Triceps	15.5	15	14.5	15
Abdomen	22	20	21	21
Thigh	18	17.5	18.5	18

Sum of skinfolds: 55 mm

$D_B = 1.099421 - (0.0009929 \times (55)) + (0.000023 \times (55)^2) - 0.0001392 \times (22)$
$D_B = 1.099421 - 0.0546095 + 0.0069575 - 0.0030624 = \underline{1.0487}$
% Fat $= ((4.57/1.0487) - 4.142 = \underline{21.6\% \text{ Fat}}$
FW $= 65 \times (0.216) = \underline{14.0 \text{ kg}}$
FFW $= 65 - 14.0 = \underline{51.0 \text{ kg}}$

Upon calculating the data, the athlete has lost 4 kg of BM which was made up of 2.6 kg of FM and lost 1.4 kg of FFM.

Laboratory Task: How Much Body Fat Do You Have?

Complete three different techniques to estimate body composition if you can.

Summary

Body composition is a valuable component of health and fitness. The techniques used include anthropometry and specific tests for estimating body composition analysis are used as descriptive measurements for coaches and trainers. Standards have been established using reference methods to determine fat- and fat-free mass. Field testing has been validated against the reference tests. Testing can be completed in the laboratory and in the field based upon the test and equipment you have at your facility. These techniques for assessing body composition range from very easy to very difficult and from least expensive to very expensive. When selecting the proper test, select the proper population-specific equation when calculating percent body fat or fat-free mass.

Body Composition - Skinfold Measurements and Calculation

Name: _____   Gender: _____

Age: _____

Body Mass (kg): _____   Height (cm): _____

Skinfold Measurements (mm)

	Trial 1	Trial 2	Trial 3	Mean
Chest	_____	_____	_____	_____
Triceps	_____	_____	_____	_____
Subscapular	_____	_____	_____	_____
Midaxillary	_____	_____	_____	_____
Suprailliac	_____	_____	_____	_____
Abdominal	_____	_____	_____	_____
Thigh	_____	_____	_____	_____
Biceps	_____	_____	_____	_____
Calf	_____	_____	_____	_____

3-site skinfold for male

Sum of chest, abdomen, and thigh skinfolds: _____ mm

3-site skinfold for female

Sum of triceps, suprailliac, and thigh skinfolds: _____ mm

Use the gender- and population-specific equations to calculate DB.

DB = _____ kg·L^{-1}

% Fat = ((4.57 / DB) – 4.142) × 100 = _____ %
(Use proper population specific formula, Table 5.1)

Fat weight (FW) = DBM × (% Fat / 100) = _____ × (_____ /
_____ /100) = _____ kg

Fat-free mass (FFM) = DBM – FW = _____ – _____ = _____ kg

Name: _____   Gender: _____

Age: _____

Body Mass (kg): _____   Height (cm): _____

Step 1: Residual Volume Determination

Vital Capacity (VC) (L): 1. _____

2. _____

3. _____

Room temperature (°C): _____
BTPS correction factor: _____

VC_{BTPS} = VC × BTPS = _____ × _____ = _____ L

Estimated RV from measurement of Residual Volume

Male Residual Volume (RV) Calculation:
Male RV = 0.24 × VC_{BTPS} _____ = _____ L

Female Residual Volume (RV) Calculation:
Female RV = 0.28 × VC_{BTPS} _____ = _____ L

Estimated Residual Volume from regression equation

Male Residual Volume (RV) Calculation:
Male RV =

Female Residual Volume (RV) Calculation:
Female RV =

Step 2: Underwater Weighing

Underwater Weighing Trials (kg)

1. _____   6. _____
2. _____   7. _____
3. _____   8. _____
4. _____   9. _____
5. _____   10. _____

Average the three highest trials (UWW): _____ kg

Dry body mass (DBM): _____ kg

Tare weight (TW): _____ kg

True underwater weight (TUWW) = UWW − TW
TUWW = _____ − _____ = _____ kg

Step 3: Body Density Equation

Water temperature (H_2O) _____ °C
Density H_2O (Table 5.3): _____

Body Volume (BV) = ((((DBM – TUWW) / DH_2O) – RV) – 0.1) = _____ L

Body Density (DB) = DBM / BV = _____ / _____ = _____ kg·L^{-1}

Step 4: Body Fat Calculation

% Fat = ((4.57 / DB) – 4.142) × 100 = _____ %
(Use proper population-specific formula, Table 5.1)

Fat weight (FW) = DBM × (% Fat/100) = _____ × (_____ / _____ / 100) = _____ kg

Fat-free mass (FFM) = DBM – FW = _____ – _____ = _____ kg

References

American College of Sports Medicine. 2021. Health-related physical fitness testing and interpretation. In: Ligouri, G. (ed). *ACSM's Guidelines for Exercise Testing and Prescription.* Wouters Kluwer.

Bazzocchi, A., Ponti, F., Albisinni, U., Battista, G. & Guglielmi, G. 2016. DXA: Technical aspects and applications. *Eur J Radiol*, 85, 1481–92.

Bergsma-Kadijk, J. A., Baumeister, B. & Deurenberg, P. 1996. Measurement of body fat in young and elderly women: Comparison between a four-compartment model and widely used reference methods. *Br J Nutr*, 75, 649–57.

Brozek, J., Grande, F., Anderson, J. T. & Keys, A. 1963. Densitometric analysis of body composition: Revision of some quantitative assumptions. *Ann N Y Acad Sci*, 110, 113–40.

Chiarlitti, N. A., Delisle-Houde, P., Reid, R. E. D., Kennedy, C. & Andersen, R. E. 2017. Importance of body composition in the National Hockey League combines physiological assessments. *J Strength Cond Res*, 32, 3135–42.

Coleman, A. E. & Lasky, L. M. 1992. Assessing running speed and body composition in professional baseball players. *J Appl Sport Sci Res*, 6, 207–13.

Collins, M. A., Millard-Stafford, M. L., Sparling, P. B., Snow, T. K., Rosskopf, L. B., Webb, S. A. & Omer, J. 1999. Evaluation of the Bod Pod for assessing body fat in collegiate football players. *Med Sci Sports Exer*, 31, 1350–6.

Cosmed, U. S. A. 2020. Bod Pod Gold Standard Body Composition Tracking System Operators Manual-P/N 210-2400, REV-I. Concord, IL.

Crapo, R. O., Morris, A. H., Clayton, P. D. & Nixon, C. R. 1982. Lung volumes in healthy nonsmoking adults. *Bull Eur Physiolpathol Respir*, 18, 419–25.

Deimel, J. F. & Dunlan, B. J. 2012. The female athlete triad. *Clin Sports Med*, 31, 247–54.

Demerath, E. W., Guo, S. S., Chumlea, W. C., Rowne, B., Roche, A. F. & Siervogel, R. M. 2002. Comparison of percent body fat estimates using air displacement plethysmography and hydrodensitometry in adults and children. *Int J Obes Relat Metab Disord*, 26, 389–96.

Evans, E. M., Rowe, D. A., Misic, M. M., Prior, B. M. & Arngrimsson, S. A. 2005. Skinfold prediction equation for athletes developed using a four-component model. *Med Sci Sports Exerc*, 37, 2006–11.

Folscher, L., Grant, G. C., Fletcher, L. & Janse van Rensberg, D. C. 2015. Ultra-marathon athletes at risk for the female athlete triad. *Sports Med – Open*, 1, 29.

Fornetti, W. C., Pivarnik, J. M., Foley, J. M. & Fiechtner, J. J. 1999. Reliability and validity of body composition measures in female athletes. *J Appl Physiol*, 87, 1114–22.

Friedl, K. E., Deluca, J. P., Marchitelli, L. J. & Vogel, J. A. 1992. Reliability of body-fat estimations from a four-compartment model by using density, body water, and bone mineral measurements. *Am J Clin Nutr*, 55, 764–70.

Fry, A. C., Kraemer, W. J., Weseman, C. A., Conroy, B. P., Gordon, S. E., Hoffman, J. R. & Maresh, C. M. 1991. The effects of an off-season strength and conditioning program on starters and non-starters in women's intercollegiate volleyball. *J Appl Sport Sci Res*, 5, 174–81.

Fryar, C. D., Carrol, M. D., Gu, Q., Afful, J. & Ogden, C. L. 2021. Anthropometric reference data for children and adults: United States, 2015–2018. *Natl Health Stat Rep, Vital Health Stat,* 3(46), 1–44.

Gibson, A. L., Wagner, D. R., & Heyward, V. H. 2019. Assessing body composition. In: Gibson, A. L., Wagner, D. R., & Heyward, V. H (eds). *Advanced Fitness Assessment and Exercise Prescription*, 8th ed. Champain, IL: Human Kinetics.

Gonzalez, A. M., Hoffman, J. R., Rogowski, J. P., Burgos, W., Manalo, E., Weise, K., Fragala, M. S. & Stout, J. R. 2013. Performance changes in NBA basketball players vary in starters vs. nonstarters over a competitive season. *J Strength Cond Res*, 27, 611–5.

Heikura, I. A., Burke, L. M., Bergland, D., Uusitalo, A. L. T., Mero, A. A. & Stellingwerff, T. 2018a. Impact of energy availability, health, and sex on hemoglobin-mass responses following live-high-train-high altitude training in elite female and male distance athletes. *Int J Sports Physiol Perform*, 13, 1090–6.

Heikura, I. A., Uusitalo, A. L. T., Stellingwerff, T., Bergland, D., Mero, A. A. & Burke, L. M. 2018b. Low energy availability is difficult. To assess but outcomes have large impact on bine injury rates in elite distance athletes. *Int J Sport Nutr Exerc Metab*, 28, 403–11.

Henricksson, P., Lof, M. & Forsum, E. 2013. Assessment and prediction of thoracic gas volume in pregnant women: An evaluation in relation to body composition assessment using air displacement plethysmography. *Br J Nutr*, 109, 111–7.

Hicks, V. L. 1992. *Validation of Near-Infrared Interactance and Skinfold Methods for Estimating Body Composition of American Indian Women [dissertation]*. Albuquerque, NM: University of New Mexico.

Houtkooper, L. B., Going, S. B., Lohman, T. G., Roche, A. F. & Van Loan, M. 1992. Bioelectrical impedance estimation of fat-free body mass in children and youth: A cross-validation study. *J Appl Physiol*, 72, 366–73.

Jackson, A. S. & Pollock, M. L. 1978. Generalized equations for predicting body density of men. *Br J Nutr*, 40, 497–504.

Jackson, A. S. & Pollock, M. L. 1985. Practical assessment of body composition. *Phys Sportsmed*, 13, 76–90.

Jackson, A. S., Pollock, M. L. & Ward, A. 1980. Generalized equations for predicting body density of women. *Med Sci Sport Exerc*, 12, 175–81.

Keay, N., Francis, G., Entwistle, I. & Hind, K. 2019. Clinical evaluation of education relating to nutrition and skeletal loading in competitive male road cyclists at risk of relative energy deficiency in sports (RED-s): 6-month randomised controlled trial. *BMJ Open Sport Exerc Med*, 5, e000523.

Kraemer, W. J., Fry, A. C., Rubin, M. R., Triplett-Mcbride, T., Gordon, S. E., Koziris, P., Lynch, J. M., Volek, J., Meuffels, S., Newton, D. E. & Fleck, R. U. 2001. Physiological and performance responses to tournament wrestling. *Med Sci Sport Exer*, 33, 1367–78.

Lifestyles Team, NHS Digital. 2020. Health survey for England 2019.

Logue, D. M., Madigan, S. M., Melin, A., Delahunt, E., Heinen, M., Mcdonnell, S. & Corish, C. A. 2020. Low energy availability in athletes 2020: An updated narrative review of prevalence, risk, within-day energy balance, knowledge, and impact on sports performance. *Nutrients*, 12, 835.

Lohman, T. G. 1986. Applicability of body composition techniques and constants for children and youths. *Exerc Sport Sci Rev*, 14, 325–57.

Lohman, T. G. 1992. *Advances in Body Composition Assessment. Current Issues in Exercise Science Series*. Monograph no. 3. Champaign, IL: Human Kinetics.

Lohman, T. G., Roche, A. F. & Martorell, R. 1988. *Anthropometric Standardization Reference Manual*. Champaign, IL: Human Kinetics.

Lohman, T. G., Harris, M., Teixeira, P. J. & Weiss, L. 2000. Assessing body composition and changes in body composition. Another look at dual-energy X-ray absorptiometry. *Ann N Y Acad Sci*, 904, 45–54.

Marra, M., Da Prat, B., Monragnese, C., Caldara, A., Sammarco, R., Pasanisi, F. & Corsetti, R. 2016. Segmental bioimpedance analysis in professional cyclists during a three week stage race. *Physiol Meas*, 37, 1035–40.

Mayhew, J. L., Piper, F. C., Schwegler, T. M. & Ball, T. E. 1989. Contributions of speed, agility, and body. Composition to anaerobic power measurements in collegiate football players. *J Appl Sport Sci Res*, 3, 101–6.

McCrory, M. A., Mole, P. A., Gomez, T. D., Dewey, K. G. & Bernauer, E. M. 1998. Body composition by air-displacement plethysmography by using predicted and measured thoracic gas volumes. *J Appl Physiol*, 84, 1475–9.

Millard-Stafford, M. L., Collins, M. A., Evans, E. M., Snow, T. K., Cureton, K. J. & Rosskopf, L. B. 2001. Use of air displacement plethysmography for estimating body fat in a four-component model. *Med Sci Sports Exerc*, 33, 1311–7.

Miller, J. M. 2016. Measured versus predicted thoracic gas volume in college students. *Med Sportiva*, XII, 2772–6.

Mitchell, H. H., Hamilton, T. S., Steggerda, F. R. & Bean, H. W. 1945. The chemical composition of the adult human body and its bearing on the biochemistry of growth. *J Bio Chem*, 158, 625–37.

Oppliger, R. A., Hielsen, D. H. & Vance, C. G. 1991. Wrestlers' minimal weight: Anthropometry, bioimpedance, and hydrostatic weighing compared. *Med Sci Sports Exerc*, 23, 247–53.

Ortiz, O., Russell, M., Daley, T. L., Baumgartner, R. N., Waki, M., Lichtman, S., Wang, J., Pierson, R. N. Jr & Heymsfield, S. B. 1992. Differences in skeletal muscle and bone mineral density between black and white females and their relevance to estimates of body composition. *Am J Clin Nutr*, 55, 8–13.

Petersen, M.R. & Hodous, T.K. 1988. Lung volume reference values for blue collar workers not exposed to occupational respiratory hazards. *J Occup Med*, 626–32.

Pietrobelli, A., Formica, C., Wang, Z. & Heymsfield, S. B. 1996. Dual-energy X-ray absorptiometry body composition model: Review of physical concepts. *Am J Physiol*, 271, E941–51.

Prior, B. M., Cureton, K. J., Modlesky, C. M., Evans, E. M., Sloniger, M. A., Saunders, M. & Lewis, R. D. 1997. In vivo validation of whole body composition estimates from dual-energy X-ray absorptiometry. *J Appl Physiol*, 83, 623–30.

Prior, B. M., Modlesky, C. M., Evans, E. M., Sloniger, M. A. & Cureton, K. J. 2001. Muscularity and the density of the fat-free mass in athletes. *J Appl. Physiol*, 90, 1523–31.

Schutte, J. E., Townsend, E. J., Hugg, J., Shoup, R. F., Malina, R. M. & Blomqvist, C. G. 1984. Density of lean body mass is greater in blacks than in whites. *J Appl Physiol Respir Environ Exerc Physiol*, 56, 1647–9.

Segal, K. R., Van Loan, M., Fitzgerald, P. I., Hodgdon, J. A. & Van Itallie, T. B. 1988. Lean body mass estimation by bioelectrical impedance analysis: A four-site cross-validation study. *Am J Clin Nutr*, 47, 7–14.

Siri, W. E. 1961. Body composition from fluid space and density. In: Brozek, J. & Henschel, A. (eds). *Techniques for Measuring Body Composition*. Natick, MA: National Academy of Sciences.

Slaughter, M. H., Lohman, T. G., Boileau, R. A., Horswill, C. A., Stillman, R. J., Van Loan, M. D. & Bemben, D. A. 1988. Skinfold equations for estimating body fatness in children and youth. *Hum Biol*, 60, 709–23.

Spehnjak, M., Gusic, M., Milnar, S., Baic, M., Andrasic, S., Selimi, M., Macak, D., Madic, D. M., Zilic Fiser, S., Sporis, G. & Trajkovic, N. 2021. Body composition in elite soccer players from youth to senior squad. *Int. J. Environ Res Public Health*, 18, 4982.

Stolarczyk, L. M., Heyward, V. H., Goodman, J. A., Grant, D. J., Kessler, K. L., Kocina, P. S. & Wilmerding, V. 1995. Predictive accuracy of bioimpedance equations in estimating fat-free mass of Hispanic women. *Med Sci Sports Exerc*, 27, 1450–6.

Vescovi, J. D., Hildebrandt, L., Miller, W. C., Hammer, R. C. & Spiller, A. 2002. Evaluation of the Bod Pod for estimating percentage fat in female collegiate athletes. *J Strength Cond Res*, 16, 599–605.

Wagner, D. R. & Heyward, V. H. 2001. Validity of two-compartment models for estimating body fat of black men. *J Appl Physiol*, 90, 649–56.

Williams, E. P., Mesidor, M., Winters, K., Dubbert, P. M. & Wyatt, S. B. 2015. Overweight and obesity: Prevalence, consequences, and causes of a growing public health problem. *Curr Obes Rep*, 4, 363–70.

Withers, R. T., Laforgia, J., & Heymsfield, S. B. 1999. Critical appraisal of the estimation of body composition via two-, three-, and four-compartment models. *Am H Hum Bill*, 11, 175–85.

6   Muscular Strength

Paul Comfort and John McMahon

Part 1: Introduction

Why Is Strength Necessary?

Strength, or the ability to exert force against an object (Suchomel et al., 2016), has been shown to be closely related to performance in numerous athletic tasks, such as sprinting (Wisloff et al., 2004; Comfort et al., 2012a; Comfort et al., 2014), change of direction (Hori et al., 2008; Nimphius et al., 2010) and jumping performance (Hori et al., 2008; Comfort et al., 2014). However, correlations do not infer cause and effect and therefore it is important to note that increases in lower body strength have been shown to result in improved performance in athletic tasks (Seitz et al., 2014; Styles et al., 2015; Comfort et al., 2019b). It is likely that the increases in sports performance are due to increased maximal force production being associated with increased rapid force production (e.g., force at specific time points [150, 200, and 250 ms]) (Comfort et al., 2019b) and rate of force development (RFD) across specific epochs (e.g., 0–100 ms, 0–200 ms) (Aagaard et al., 2002; Andersen and Aagaard, 2006; Andersen et al., 2010). An increase in force produced over a specific duration results in an increase in impulse (impulse = force × time), and impulse determines acceleration. Therefore, increased impulse results in greater acceleration and also a higher movement velocity.

Low strength levels have been shown to be a strong predictor of injury risk (Malone et al., 2019), with strength training reducing sports injuries by >30% and overuse injuries by ~50% (Lauersen et al., 2014). Interestingly, based on the results of their meta-analysis, Lauersen et al. (2018) reported that when volume and intensity were *appropriately progressed*, injury risks were reduced. It is unsurprising that strength training reduces the risk of musculoskeletal injuries as the associated tissue (e.g., muscles, tendons, and bones) adaptations improve the ability of these structures to tolerate increased loads. In addition, increased strength has also been shown to improve rapid force production (Aagaard et al., 2002; Andersen and Aagaard, 2006; Comfort et al., 2022), which may be required in order to correct adverse sporting movement patterns especially when decelerating on landing from a jump, during changes of direction, and in response to collisions.

Why Assess Strength?

It is important to periodically assess strength (e.g., repetition maximum testing [RM]); both to determine the magnitude of change which has occurred in response to training and competition and to enable appropriate loads to be selected for

DOI: 10.4324/9781003186762-6

the subsequent training phase, as the load/intensity of resistance training has been shown to be responsible for specific muscle fibre adaptations (Fry, 2004). However, while RM testing makes determining the recommended training loads for specific exercises easy, it provides no insight into how the force was applied. In contrast, during isometric assessments, it is possible to determine not only maximal force production, but also how rapidly force can be produced, which may be more sensitive to changes than maximal strength or force production, especially during periods of intensive training and/or competition (Hornsby et al., 2017; Suarez et al., 2019).

How Do Different Methods of Assessing Strength/Force Compare?

The terms strength and force tend to be used interchangeably; however, it is essential to understand the differences between the two terms and how they can be assessed. Strength is usually assessed during dynamic tasks, for example, when evaluating the loads lifted during RM testing. In this case, however, ≤6RM should be classed as strength, whereas higher repetition ranges, such as a 10RM should be considered strength endurance. It is also worth noting that while predicting 1RM performance from other RM performances is possible (e.g., predicting 1RM from 6RM performance), there is greater error and variability as the number of repetitions increases (Morales and Sobonya, 1996; Julio et al., 2012).

While force-time variables assessed during single joint isometric assessments, such as the knee extension, are highly reliable, they do not relate well to performance in athletic tasks (Blackburn and Morrissey, 1998). In contrast to single-joint isometric assessments, force-time variables assessed during multi-joint assessment, such as the isometric mid-thigh pull (IMTP), demonstrate strong to almost perfect correlations with dynamic strength measures (e.g., 1RM squat, deadlift clean, and snatch) and measures of athletic performance (e.g., short sprint and change of direction) (Comfort et al., 2019a) (Figure 6.1). The assessment of maximal force and rapid force production characteristics (e.g., force at specific time points [100 ms, 150 ms, 200 ms, and 250 ms], RFD and impulse over specific epochs [0–100 ms, 0–200 ms]) are usually assessed during isometric assessments, with the time-constrained variables (Figure 6.2) more sensitive to acute changes (e.g., reductions when fatigued) than peak force (Hornsby et al., 2017; Suarez et al., 2019).

Part 2: Why Perform Isometric Strength Assessments

As already mentioned, multi-joint isometric assessments, such as the IMTP and isometric squat can provide additional insight regarding how quickly force can be produced, either in terms of force at specific time points (e.g., force at 100-, 150-, 200- and 250 ms) or RFD and impulse across specific epochs (e.g., 0-150 ms, 0-250 ms), which may are sensitive to changes than peak force, especially during periods of intensive training and/or competition (Hornsby et al., 2017; Suarez et al., 2019). Additionally, as athletic tasks are time-constrained, time-related force-time variables may be more indicative of how changes in force production characteristics, as a result of training and competition may affect performance in athletic tasks.

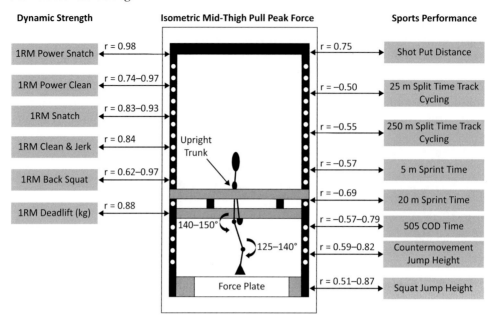

Figure 6.1 Relationships between isometric mid-thigh (IMTP) pull peak force and performance in other tasks. (Adapted from Comfort et al., 2019a].)

How Do Different Assessment Methods Compare?

While there are clear similarities in the IMTP and isometric squat in terms of the key principles of isometric assessments, including sampling frequency (recommendations 1000 Hz) (Dos'Santos et al., 2016), contraction duration (5 seconds), cueing (push as fast and hard as possible), and maintenance of an upright trunk (5–10° forward lean) with hip angles of 125–150° (Brady et al., 2018b; Haff, 2019; Comfort et al., 2019a), there are clear differences. One key difference between tests is the commonly

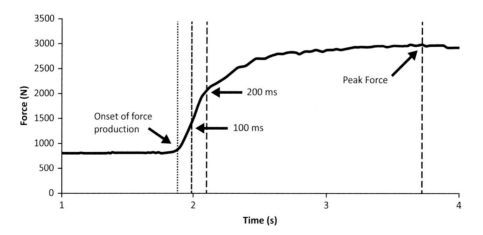

Figure 6.2 Illustration of identification of force at 100 ms and 200 ms, which can be used to calculate mean RFD across specific epochs.

used knee joint angles with greater knee flexion in the isometric squat compared to the IMTP. The recommendations for the IMTP knee angles are 125–145° (Comfort et al., 2019a), while the commonly reported range for the isometric squat is 90–120° (Brady et al., 2018b; Haff, 2019), which may explain some of the differences in force-time characteristics between the two tests. In general, the peak force is higher during the isometric squat, whereas rapid force production (i.e., force at specific time points, RFD) tends to be higher during the IMTP (Nuzzo et al., 2008; Brady et al., 2018a; Brady et al., 2018b).

Additionally, there are distinct differences in how the force-time data is analysed between studies, as well as between multi-joint isometric tests. One of these important differences, especially in relation to time-related variables, is the identification of the onset of force production, including manual identification, arbitrary thresholds (e.g., 20 N, 40 N), relative thresholds (e.g., 5% body mass), and relative thresholds taking into account system (athlete and force plate) noise and force fluctuation using 5 standard deviations of body mass during a period of quiet standing (Dos'Santos et al., 2017a; Brady et al., 2018a). In addition, there are numerous differences in the methods used to calculate RFD, including peak and mean RFD, RFD across specific epochs (e.g., 0–100 ms, 0–200 ms, and 100–200 ms), and the use of moving average windows, with Haff et al. (2015) recommending the use of RFD across pre-determined epochs, rather than peak RFD. Standardization of the onset threshold and the procedures for calculating RFD are essential for longitudinal evaluation of force production, or when attempting to compare performances between groups/studies.

Isometric Mid-Thigh Pull

Athletes should complete a standard generalized warm-up of body weight squats and lunges and the dynamic mid-thigh pull at submaximal loads. This should be followed by submaximal trials of the IMTP, e.g., 3–5 second effort at ~50% maximal effort, ~75% maximal effort, ~90% maximal effort, separated by a 60-second rest, which can be considered as part of the familiarization process (Comfort et al., 2019a). During this time, the athlete should be secured to the bar using lifting straps and athletic tape to ensure that grip strength is not a limiting factor (Haff et al., 1997; Haff et al., 2005).

Prior to initiation of IMTP trials the bar height should be adjusted to ensure the correct body position that replicates the start of the second pull position during the clean. The bar height should then be adjusted up or down to allow the athlete to obtain the optimal knee (125–145°) and hip (140–150°) angles (Beckham et al., 2012; Beckham et al., 2018; Dos'Santos et al., 2017b) (Figure 6.1). The body position should be very similar to the second pull of the clean and the clean grip mid-thigh pull exercise (DeWeese et al., 2013): upright torso, slight flexion in the knee resulting in clear dorsiflexion, shoulder girdle retracted and depressed, shoulders slightly behind the vertical plane of the bar, feet centred under the bar approximately hip-width apart, knees in front of the bar, and the bar in contact with the thighs (close to the inguinal crease dependent on limb lengths) (Figure 6.3) (Comfort et al., 2019a).

While the use of a "self-selected" body position, which represents the start of the second pull of the clean, is likely beneficial to efficiency of testing, it is not recommended without ensuring that the hip and knee joint angles fall within the ranges recommended earlier, due to the influence of body positioning on force generation (Beckham et al., 2012; Beckham et al., 2018; Dos'Santos et al., 2017b). The bar height

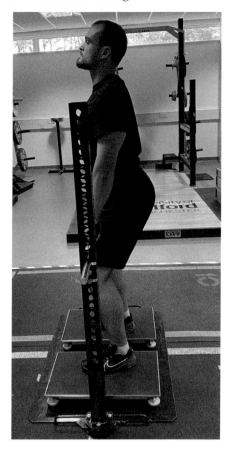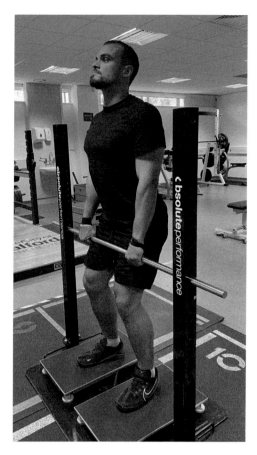

Figure 6.3 Example posture for the IMTP (upright trunk = 5–10° forward lean, resulting in a hip angle of 140–150°; dorsiflexed ankle; knee angle of 125–140°; representing the start of the second pull of a clean).

used and joint angles obtained should be recorded so that repeated measurements can be standardized and therefore replicate the individuals' body position between sessions, ensuring that differing results in subsequent testing are not the result of changed body position (Beckham et al., 2018; Dos'Santos et al., 2017b). Sufficient pre-tension to achieve the correct body position and remove "slack" from the body, but without any more pre-tension than is necessary to get the "quiet standing" necessary for a stable force baseline (Maffiuletti et al., 2016). The baseline force during the period of quiet standing should represent body mass with minimal fluctuation, with trials where a change in force >50 N occurs during this period of quiet standing rejected (Dos'Santos et al., 2017a). This should be explained to each athlete and they should be encouraged to stay as still as possible during this period to accurately determine body weight and onset threshold (e.g., an increase in force >5 standard deviations of the force during the period of quiet standing) (Comfort et al., 2019a).

Standardized instructions should be given to the athlete, such as "push your feet into the ground as fast and as hard as possible," to ensure that both maximal RFD and PF are obtained (Bemben et al., 1990; Halperin et al., 2016). It is essential

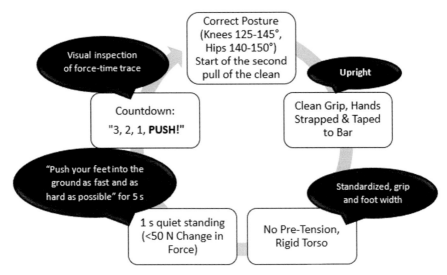

Acceptable trials: <250 N difference in peak force, minimal pre-tension (<50N) with force representing body mass, no countermovement at the start

Figure 6.4 Standardized IMTP Testing Procedure. (Adapted from Comfort et al., 2019a].)

that athletes understand that the focus is to drive the feet directly into the force platform and not attempt to pull the bar with the arms or rise up onto their toes (Comfort et al., 2019a). A countdown of "3, 2, 1, PUSH!" gives the athlete sufficient warning to be ready to give maximum effort and should provide at least one second of quiet standing prior to the onset of the pull (Figure 6.4). Cueing to "push" rather than "pull" helps emphasize the fact that the athletes should be pushing with their legs and not pulling with their arms, attempting to drive their feet into the force plates.

A minimum of two trials should be collected, provided that each of those trials has no errors by the athlete (e.g., countermovement, excessive pre-tension, leaning on the bar prior to the pull). If PF increases between trials, additional trials should be performed until the PF values of the trials are separated by <250 N (Haff et al., 1997; Haff et al., 2005).

Visual inspection of the force-time curves during testing can easily be used to determine if the trials are acceptable, or if additional trials should be performed. In addition to the trials being within 250 N between attempts, trials should be repeated if there is not a stable weighing period (clear fluctuation in the force-time data) or a clear countermovement prior to the initiation of the pull (Figure 6.5), as this will interfere with accurate identification of the initiation of the pull (19), or if the PF occurs at the end of the trial.

Data Analysis

Figure 6.5 illustrates an acceptable force-time curve, with >1 second of quiet standing, which represents the athlete's body mass, with no countermovement (decrease in force prior to an increase in force), which permits the use of the threshold of an increase in force which is >5 standard deviations above the force during the period

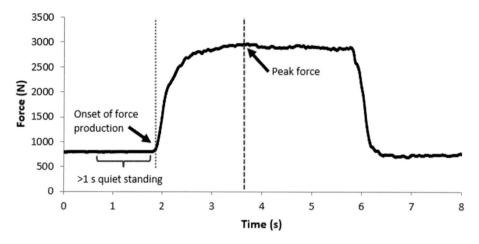

Figure 6.5 Acceptable force-time data, including at least one second of quiet standing that represents body weight, no countermovement and peak force occurring within two seconds of the start of force production.

of quiet standing. Additionally, the peak force also occurs in <2 seconds of the onset of the pull. It is important to note, however, that if calculating RFD, this should not be the change in force/change in time between the onset and peak force (Figure 6.6), as this dramatically alters the slope of the mean RFD curve, compared to the actual slope of the curve if calculated RFD as the mean across specific epochs (Figure 6.2).

If using force-plate-specific software, which does not permit the use of the threshold identified earlier, but instead uses an arbitrary threshold (e.g., 20 N), it is essential to make sure that the residual noise and the force during the period of quiet standing do not exceed this threshold, as this will result in early identification of the start of the pull. In such instances, it may be possible to alter the arbitrary thresholds used;

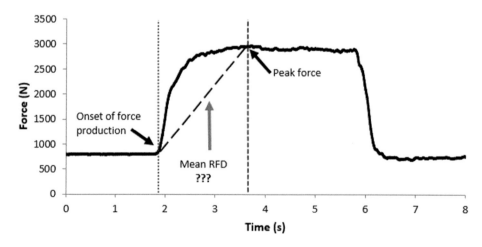

Figure 6.6 Illustration of why mean RFD should not be calculated from the onset of force production to the peak force, as the mean RFD slope is not representative of the slope of the force-time curve.

however, this should be standardized between testing sessions to ensure that any time-specific variables are comparable for longitudinal comparisons.

Data Interpretation for Multi-Joint Isometric Assessments

Ideally, isometric force data should be reported as a net force, rather than gross force, as gross force includes the athletes' mass, which benefits heavier athletes. It is worth considering both absolute and relative (ratio scaled) force production, with relative performances permitting appropriate comparisons between athletes of different statures (Comfort and Pearson, 2014; Suchomel et al., 2018) and between sexes (Nimphius, 2018; Nimphius, 2019). To calculate relative force, simply divide the absolute performance by body mass, whether assessing peak force or force at specific time points:

$$Relative\ Strength = \frac{Absolute\ Force}{Body\ Mass}$$

It is suggested that relative net force and force at specific time points are evaluated, to determine the athletes' maximum force-generating capacity and how much of their maximum force they can express rapidly. To achieve this expressing force at 150-, 200- and 250 ms as a percentage of peak force may be advantageous (Comfort et al., 2019b). If peak force is considered good or excellent (Table 6.1), but only a low percentage of peak force can be generated across the aforementioned time points, then it would be pertinent to emphasize more ballistic and plyometric styles of training, whereas if a high percentage of peak force can be generated at 150-, 200-, and 250 ms, greater emphasis should be placed on increasing maximal force production.

Laboratory Task

Collect some IMTP data, following the protocols described earlier and then determine how you would categorize your performance, based on the values in Table 6.1.

Isometric Squat

Some practitioners, researchers, and athletes have preferences regarding the use/performance of the IMTP and isometric squat; however, when posture is comparable, there is little difference in the outputs obtained from the two tests. In general, the

Table 6.1 Recommendations for interpretation of relative peak force categories.

Interpretation	Relative Peak Force
Excellent	>50.0 N/kg
Good	40.0–49.9 N/kg
Average	30.0–39.9 N/kg
Below Average	<30 N/kg

* These data should be considered as descriptive and not normative. It would be worth determining the normative data for your particular sport and level of competition

isometric squat results in slightly higher forces, whereas the IMTP results in slightly higher RFD and force at specific time points. Numerous postures have been used for isometric squat testing, with knee flexion varying notably across studies, ranging from 90–125° (Drake et al., 2017; Brady et al., 2018b; Haff, 2019; Drake et al., 2019a), while an upright trunk is always reported and should always be adopted. Differences in posture affect the resultant force-time characteristics and therefore should be standardized between testing sessions and carefully considered when comparing data to that presented in published studies, or normative data.

As with the IMTP, a general warm-up should be performed, followed by submaximal trials of the isometric squat, e.g., 3–5-second effort at ~50% maximal effort, ~75% maximal effort, ~90% maximal effort, separated by a 60-second rest. During these trials, it is essential to watch the athlete to determine if posture is appropriate and maintained throughout. Subsequently, the force-time data should be visually inspected to identify any technical errors that occur, such as an initial countermovement, or peak force occurring at the end of the trial.

Figure 6.7 summarizes the sequence of isometric squat testing. The knee joint angle should be measured using a goniometer and standardized between testing sessions. It is worth noting that RFD values during such testing have been reported not to meet an acceptable level, although the highest force is achieved during this procedure.

An alternative "explosive" isometric squat procedure (Figure 6.8) has been recommended by Drake et al. (2019b), which has been shown to substantially improve the reliability of RFD compared to the traditional procedure described earlier. The key differences are the duration of the maximal effort (e.g., traditional = 5 seconds vs. *explosive* = 1 second) and the coaching cue (e.g., traditional = "push as **HARD** and fast as possible" vs. *explosive* = "push as **FAST** and hard as possible"). While the "explosive" isometric squat procedure results in much more reliable RFD, peak force

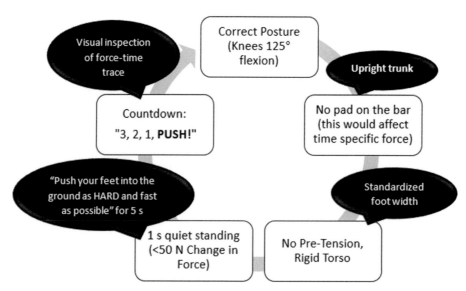

Acceptable trials: <250 N difference in peak force, minimal pre-tension (<50N) with force representing body mass, no countermovement at the start

Figure 6.7 Standardized traditional isometric squat testing procedure.

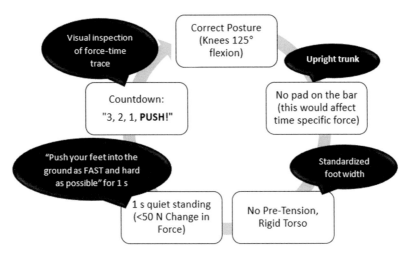

Acceptable trials: <250 N difference in peak force, minimal pre-tension (<50N) with force representing body mass, no countermovement at the start

Figure 6.8 Standardized "explosive" isometric squat testing procedure.

is much lower when compared with the traditional protocol. As such, for isometric squat testing, if peak force and RFD are to be monitored, it would be advisable to perform three trials of the explosive isometric squat followed by three trials of the traditional isometric squat.

Laboratory Task

Collect data using the traditional and *"explosive"* versions of the isometric squat and see how the relative peak force, force at specific time points, and RFD values compare, using Table 6.2.

Part 3: Dynamic Assessments

Dynamic assessments of strength are great for determining appropriate loads for specific exercises, and can be included within training sessions, as appropriate. For example, if evaluating the progressing from a general strength phase of training, where the athletes have been performing multiple sets of 5–6 repetitions (usually with 1–2

Table 6.2 Comparison of force-time characteristics between methods of isometric squat testing.

Variable	Traditional	"Explosive"
Relative Peak Force		
Force at 150 ms		
Force at 200 ms		
Force at 250 ms		
RFD 0–150 ms		
RFD 0–200 ms		
RFD 0–250 ms		
RFD = rate of force development		

repetitions in reserve for each set), a 5RM or 3RM could be performed during key exercises towards the start of a training session at the end of a meso-cycle. It is also worth noting that while predicting 1RM performance from other RM performances is possible (e.g., predicting 1RM from 6RM performance), there is greater error and variability as the number of repetitions increases (Morales and Sobonya, 1996; Julio et al., 2012).

Where possible, 1RM assessments are advised due to the very high reliability (Grgic et al., 2020) even in inexperienced lifters (Comfort and McMahon, 2015) and youth athletes (Faigenbaum et al., 2012), with measurement error and smallest detectable differences of only ~5% (Comfort and McMahon, 2015). In comparison, prediction from other RM ranges or from load velocity profiles tend to result in errors of >10% (Morales and Sobonya, 1996; Julio et al., 2012; Banyard et al., 2017; Sayers et al., 2018; Fernandes et al., 2021).

General Repetition Maximum Testing Protocols

The general principles and protocols for 5 RM testing are the same irrespective of exercise, including an exercise specific warm-up, which must be non-fatiguing, followed by RM attempts. After the initial RM attempt, the load should be increased by 2.5–5.0% depending on the athletes' perceived effort during the previous attempt. The magnitude of the increase in load can also be informed by the observed velocity and technique during the final repetition. A rest period of 3–5 minutes should be provided between attempts to minimize any cumulative fatigue due to lactic acid accumulation and phosphor-creatine depletion (Figure 6.9). The 5RM should be achieved,

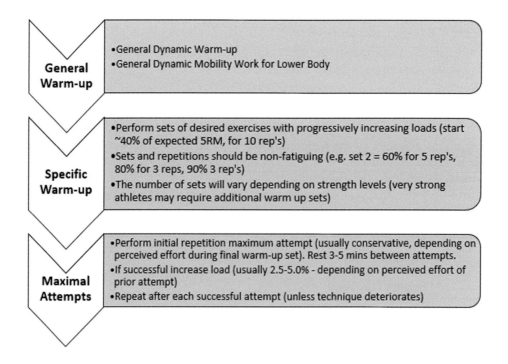

Figure 6.9 Example flow diagram of 5 repetitions' maximum testing.

ideally, within 3 attempts, to minimize the level of fatigue. If the 5RM is not achieved within 3 attempts, it would be advisable to repeat the attempts, starting at a higher load, after 48–72 hours. Specific guidance for bench press, back squat, and power clean is provided later.

Similar to the 5RM general principles and protocols for 1RM testing being the same irrespective of exercise, including an exercise-specific warm-up, which must be non-fatiguing (for power-based exercises, the warm-up repetitions should ideally be performed in a cluster set format), followed by RM attempts. After the initial 1RM attempt, the load should be increased by 2.5–5.0% depending on the athletes' perceived effort during the previous attempt. The magnitude of the increase in load can also be informed by the observed velocity and technique during the previous attempt (Note: If technique is not safe, testing should be terminated). A rest period of 3–5 minutes should be provided between attempts to minimize any cumulative fatigue due to lactic acid accumulation and phosphor-creatine depletion (Figure 6.9). The 5RM should be achieved, ideally, within 5 attempts, to minimize the level of fatigue. If the 1RM is not achieved within 5 attempts, it would be advisable to repeat the attempts, starting at a higher load, after 48–72 hours. Specific guidance for bench press, back squat, and power clean are provided later.

Set-up of equipment and performance of the test must be carefully considered for both safety and to ensure that procedures are standardized and changes in performance are a result of adaptations not change in procedures.

Bench Press

The bench should be set so that the bar is resting on supports close to arm's length, ideally with safety pins set at the bottom position, just below where the bar would touch the chest when a full inhalation has been completed, and also that the safety pins will take the weight of the barbell if the athlete exhales just in case failure occurs. A spotter (or multiple spotters [one behind the athlete and one at either end of the barbell] if the athlete is strong) should be used to assist the athlete in lifting the bar off the rack and moving into the "start" position, and then to assist in replacing the bar back on to the rack after the repetition(s) have been completed. The spotter(s) are also there in case the athlete fails the lift, to assist with safely returning the barbell to the rack. The spotters should not touch barbell while the athlete is performing the lift unless the athlete indicates that they require assistance. If there are multiple spotters, the spotters at either end of the barbell should communicate effectively, if required, to lift the bar, to ensure that it is lifted symmetrically.

The athlete should set up on the bench so that their feet are in contact with the floor, buttocks, and shoulder blades in contact with the bench, with no excessive arch in the lower back (unlike the bench press style adopted by powerlifters, where the arch in the back is exaggerated) and the barbell positioned on the rack above their eyes. Grip width should be standardized so that the outside part of the hands are ~1.5 × biacromial width (Green and Comfort, 2007). When the athlete and spotter lift the barbell off the rack, the barbell should be repositioned above the athlete's chest, with the athlete's arms fully extended. The spotter should keep contact with the bar until the athlete indicates that they have control.

Once warmed up and the maximal attempts commence, the athlete should initiate the descent phase of the lift in a controlled manner, aiming for the bar to touch the bottom of the sternum, resulting in ~45° angle between the humerus and the trunk. There should be a brief pause when the bar reached the sternum, ensuring that the bar does not bounce off of the chest, followed by a forceful, yet controlled, extension of the arms until the barbell returns back to the starting position. Once the desired number of repetitions is completed (e.g., 1 repetition during the 1RM, or 5 repetitions during the 5RM), the spotter should assist with guiding the barbell back to the rack.

Back Squat

Ideally, the back squat should be performed in a power rack/squat rack, with the safety bars set just below (~3–4 cm) the desired squat depth (ideally so that the thighs are parallel with the floor and the inguinal crease of the hip reaches the same height as the top of the knee), in case the athlete fails the lift, or loses control on the descent phase. The athlete should also be instructed on how to safely drop/lower the weight onto the safety bars during a failed attempt. If squat stands are being used, as a power rack/squat rack is unavailable, the athlete should be familiar with the technique of safely dropping the weight during a failed attempt. If the athlete is not familiar with or competent at safely dropping the weight and only squat stands are available, it is advisable not to perform a maximal squat test until appropriate equipment is available, or the athlete is competent.

The bar should be positioned on the rack at a height which permits the athlete to lift the barbell out of the rack without plantar flexing. The athlete should position the barbell on the trapezius, in a high bar position, taking a grip ~1.5 × biacromial width, if shoulder flexibility permits, as this aids with the maintenance of an extended rather than flexed thoracic spine. The athlete's feet should both be positioned under the barbell (not adopting a lunge position), and the knees and hips should be extended so that the bar is lifted from the rack, followed by 2 small steps backwards, to clear the hooks on the rack. The athlete does not need to be a great distance from the rack, as the barbell should move in a vertical path and therefore should not be at risk of catching on the hooks of the rack.

The athlete should adopt a natural foot position, usually hip to shoulder width apart, with the feet in a naturally orientated position, usually externally rotated 15–30° (Comfort et al., 2018). This position along with squat depth (ideally so that the thighs are parallel with the floor and the inguinal crease of the hip reaches the same height as the top of the knee; however, if working with weightlifters' full depth would be a better option) should be standardized between testing sessions to ensure a consistent range of motion and therefore displacement of the barbell. The athlete should initiate the descent phase of the lift in a controlled manner (performing the Valsalva manoeuvre if a 1RM attempt) until the desired depth is reached, at which point they should forcefully and simultaneously extend the hips and knees while maintaining spinal alignment, until full extension is achieved. The athlete should then walk forward and plate the barbell safely back on the rack.

Power Clean

It is essential that the athlete performs the power clean with good technique, as determined by an appropriately qualified strength and conditioning coach. A detailed description of correct power clean technique is beyond the scope of this chapter, although key points will be highlighted: for more detail on correct power clean technique and coaching progressions, see Verhoeff et al. (2020). In the start position, the athlete's hips should be slightly higher than the knees with the shoulders in front of the barbell while maintaining a neutral spine. The bar should initially be lifting in a controlled manner during the first pull phase, via extension of the knees, while maintaining a neutral spine. Once the transition phase commences, there should be a clear acceleration of the barbell, as the athlete's knees move over the toes and the trunk moves into an upright position, which should fluidly progress into the second pull phase, where there is a rapid extension of hips, knees, and ankles, and the barbell reaches its peak vertical velocity. Once full extension is achieved, the athlete should rapidly flex the hips and knees to drop into a shallow front squat position (the knees should achieve no more than 90° flexion), with the elbows high and the barbell received on the anterior deltoids, while ensuring that there is no flexion in the spine. From this point, the athletes should extend knees and hips until they reach a standing position, where, once stable, they should drop the barbell onto the lifting platform.

Data Analysis and Interpretation

It is worth considering both absolute and relative (ratio scaled) performances, with relative performances permitting appropriate comparisons between athletes of different statures (Comfort and Pearson, 2014; Suchomel et al., 2018) and between sexes (Nimphius, 2018; Nimphius, 2019). To calculate relative performance, simply divide the absolute performance by body mass:

$$Relative\ Strength = \frac{Absolute\ Strength}{Body\ Mass}$$

It is best not to consider maximal strength in isolation, but also in comparison to performances in other tasks, such as short sprint and jump performance. For example, if an athlete demonstrates a good relative back squat performance (Table 6.3), but a low countermovement jump height and a substandard 20 m sprint time, it is likely that rapid force production rather than maximal force production should be emphasized during the next phase of training, along with some refinement in sprint and jump technique. In contrast, if the athlete demonstrates an excellent countermovement jump height and 20 m sprint time, but has below average relative

Table 6.3 Recommended relative strength categories.

Interpretation	Bench Press	Back Squat	Power Clean
Excellent	>1.5 kg/kg	>2.0 kg/kg	>1.5 kg/kg
Good	1.2–1.5 kg/kg	1–7–2.0 kg/kg	1.2–1.5 kg/kg
Average	0.8–1.2 kg/kg	1.4–1.7 kg/kg	0.8–1.2 kg/kg
Below Average	<0.8 kg/kg	<1.4 kg/kg	<0.8 kg/kg

* These data should be considered as descriptive and not normative. It would be worth determining the normative data for your particular sport and level of competition

back squat strength, it is likely that they are technically proficient at jumping and sprinting and can express their strength rapidly, highlighting the need to increase relative strength.

Laboratory Task

Compare your performances in some of these 1RM tasks to the data in Table 6.3 to identify areas where you may benefit from strength development. Also compare your relative performances in the dynamic strength assessments to the performances you achieved in the isometric assessments. Finally, as isometric force production is commonly reported to be closely associated with maximal strength, perform some correlations to see if the data from yourself and your peers demonstrate associations similar to those presented in Figure 6.1.

Velocity-Based Predictions of 1 Repetition Maximum

While proponents of velocity-based methods commonly state that there are fluctuations in 1RM performance across days which should be considered when prescribing training loads, there is no empirical evidence to substantiate this concept or any quantification of this magnitude. In fact, maximum strength and force production tends to be quite stable, even during periods of high intensity and high-volume training (Hornsby et al., 2017; Suarez et al., 2019). Banyard et al. (2017) also demonstrated much higher reliability and much lower measurement error in 1RM performance compared to velocity-based predictions from submaximal loads. While some authors report low magnitudes of error through prediction equations when expressed as a percentage error, these can be substantial. For example, Caven et al. (2020) a very large to almost perfect correlation (r = 0.76–0.97) between 1RM bench press and prediction from both multiple (eight loads) and two-point (two loads) load velocity predictions. However, while they reported an error range of 2.1–3.4 kg when predicting 1RM bench press, this equates to an average error of nearly 10%, with individuals demonstrating overestimations of ~12 kg, which could be as much as 25% error, although the specific percentage error rates were not provided. Similarly, Fernandes et al. (2021) reported errors in predicting 1RM performance from load-velocity profiles of 8.2–20.4% in the bench press, 8.6–19.9% in the bent-over-row and 5.7–17.0% in the squat. Therefore, based on current load-velocity profiles, it may be best to avoid predicting 1RM performances, as errors of 10–20% 1RM could easily result in inappropriate loads being selected during training, which may either result in loads that are too low to elicit the desired adaptations or expose the athlete to unnecessary loads which may increase injury risk.

Summary

It is extremely important to accurately monitor changes in strength and force production, in response to training, to evaluate the effectiveness of the previous phase of training and inform subsequent phases of training. Consideration of measurement error (see Chapter 4 for more on this) and the magnitude of change that highlights a meaningful change are of utmost importance. In addition, such assessments are not required on a daily basis but rather at the start/end of specific phases of training. It is also important not to consider these assessments in isolation, but in conjunction with other assessments of the athlete's physical capabilities as part of a holistic testing battery, which should be used in conjunction with an appropriate needs analysis of the athlete's sport, to enable appropriate and informed programming priorities to be made.

References

Aagaard, P., Simonsen, E. B., Andersen, J. L., Magnusson, P. & Dyhre-Poulsen, P. 2002. Increased rate of force development and neural drive of human skeletal muscle following resistance training. *J Appl Physiol*, 93, 1318–26.

Andersen, L. L. & Aagaard, P. 2006. Influence of maximal muscle strength and intrinsic muscle contractile properties on contractile rate of force development. *Eur J Appl Physiol*, 96, 46–52.

Andersen, L. L., Andersen, J. L., Zebis, M. K. & Aagaard, P. 2010. Early and late rate of force development: Differential adaptive responses to resistance training? *Scand J Med Sci Sports*, 20, e162–9.

Banyard, H. G., Nosaka, K. & Haff, G. G. 2017. Reliability and validity of the Load–Velocity relationship to predict the 1RM back squat. *J Strength Cond Res*, 31.

Beckham, G., Lamont, H., Sato, K., Ramsey, M., Haff, G. G. & Stone, M. 2012. Isometric strength of powerlifters in key positions of the conventional deadlift. *J Trainol*, 1.

Beckham, G. K., Sato, K., Mizuguchi, S., Haff, G. G. & Stone, M. H. 2018. Effect of body position on force production during the isometric mid-thigh pull. *J Strength Cond Res*, 32(1), 48–56.

Bemben, M. G., Clasey, J. L. & Massey, B. H. 1990. The effect of the rate of muscle contraction on the force-time curve parameters of male and female subjects. *Res Q Exerc Sport*, 61, 96–9.

Blackburn, J. R. & Morrissey, M. C. 1998. The relationship between open and closed kinetic chain strength of the lower limb and jumping performance. *J Orthop Sports Phys Ther*, 27, 430–5.

Brady, C. J., Harrison, A. J. & Comyns, T. M. 2018a. A review of the reliability of biomechanical variables produced during the isometric mid-thigh pull and isometric squat and the reporting of normative data. *Sports Biomech*, 1–25.

Brady, C. J., Harrison, A. J., Flanagan, E. P., Haff, G. G. & Comyns, T. M. 2018b. A comparison of the isometric midthigh pull and isometric squat: Intraday reliability, usefulness, and the magnitude of difference between tests. *Int J Sports Physiol Perform*, 13, 844–52.

Caven, E. J. G., Bryan, T. J. E., Dingley, A. F., Drury, B., Garcia-Ramos, A., Perez-Castilla, A., Arede, J. & Fernandes, J. F. T. 2020. Group versus individualised minimum velocity thresholds in the prediction of maximal strength in trained female athletes. *Int J Environ Res Public Health*, 17.

Comfort, P. & McMahon, J. J. 2015. Reliability of maximal back squat and power clean performances in inexperienced athletes. *J Strength Cond Res*, 29, 3089–96.

Comfort, P., Bullock, N. & Pearson, S. J. 2012a. A comparison of maximal squat strength and 5-, 10-, and 20-meter sprint times, in athletes and recreationally trained men. *J Strength Cond Res*, 26, 937–40.

Comfort, P., Dos'Santos, T., Beckham, G. K., Stone, M. H., Guppy, S. N. & Haff, G. G. 2019a. Standardization and methodological considerations for the isometric mid-thigh pull. *Strength Cond J*, 41, 57–79.

Comfort, P., Dos'Santos, T., Jones, P. A., McMahon, J. J., Suchomel, T. J., Bazyler, C. & Stone, M. H. 2019b. Normalization of early isometric force production as a percentage of peak force during multijoint isometric assessment. *Int J Sports Physiol Perform*, 15, 478–82.

Comfort, P., Haigh, A. & Matthews, M. J. 2012b. Are changes in maximal squat strength during preseason training reflected in changes in sprint performance in Rugby league players? *J Strength Cond Res*, 26, 772–6.

Comfort, P., Jones, P. A., Thomas, C., Dos'Santos, T., McMahon, J. J. & Suchomel, T. J. 2022. Changes in early and maximal isometric force production in response to moderate- and high-load strength and power training. *J Strength Cond Res*, 36, 593–9.

Comfort, P., McMahon, J. J. & Suchomel, T. J. 2018. Optimizing squat technique—Revisited. *Strength Cond J*, 40, 68–74.

Comfort, P. & Pearson, S. J. 2014. Scaling–which methods best predict performance? *J Strength Cond Res*, 28, 1565–72.

Comfort, P., Stewart, A., Bloom, L. & Clarkson, B. 2014. Relationships between strength, sprint, and jump performance in well-trained youth soccer players. *J Strength Cond Res*, 28, 173–7.

DeWeese, B. H., Serrano, A. J., Scruggs, S. K. & Burton, J. D. 2013. The midthigh pull: Proper application and progressions of a weightlifting movement derivative. *Strength Cond J*, 35, 54–8.

Dos'Santos, T., Jones, P. A., Comfort, P. & Thomas, C. 2017a. Effect of different onset thresholds on isometric mid-thigh pull force-time variables. *J Strength Cond Res*, 31, 3467–73.

Dos'Santos, T., Jones, P. A., Kelly, J., McMahon, J. J., Comfort, P. & Thomas, C. 2016. Effect of sampling frequency on isometric midthigh-pull kinetics. *Int J Sports Physiol Perform*, 11, 255–60.

Dos'Santos, T., Thomas, C., Jones, P. A., McMahon, J. J. & Comfort, P. 2017b. The effect of hip joint angle on isometric mid-thigh pull kinetics. *J Strength Cond Res*, Publish 31(10), 2748–57.

Drake, D., Kennedy, R. & Wallace, E. 2017. The validity and responsiveness of isometric lower body multi-joint tests of muscular strength: A systematic review. *Sports Med – Open*, 3, 23.

Drake, D., Kennedy, R. A. & Wallace, E. S. 2019a. Measuring what matters in isometric multi-joint rate of force development. *J Sports Sci*, 37, 2667–75.

Drake, D., Kennedy, R. A. & Wallace, E. S. 2019b. Multi-joint rate of force development testing protocol affects reliability and the smallest detectible difference. *J Sports Sci*, 37, 1570–81.

Faigenbaum, A. D., Mcfarland, J. E., Herman, R. E., Naclerio, F., Ratamess, N. A., Kang, J. & Myer, G. D. 2012. Reliability of the one-repetition-maximum power clean test in adolescent athletes. *J Strength Cond Res*, 26, 432–7.

Fernandes, J. F. T., Dingley, A. F., Garcia-Ramos, A., Perez-Castilla, A., Tufano, J. J. & Twist, C. 2021. Prediction of one repetition maximum using reference minimum velocity threshold values in young and middle-aged resistance-trained males. *Behav Sci (Basel, Switzerland)*, 11, 71.

Fry, A. C. 2004. The role of resistance exercise intensity on muscle fibre adaptations. *Sports Med*, 34, 663–79.

Green, C. M. & Comfort, P. 2007. The affect of grip width on bench press performance and risk of injury. *Strength Cond J*, 29, 10–4.

Grgic, J., Lazinica, B., Schoenfeld, B. J. & Pedisic, Z. 2020. Test-retest reliability of the one-repetition maximum (1RM) strength assessment: A systematic review. *Sports Med Open*, 6, 31.

Haff, G. G., Stone, M., O'bryant, H. S., Harman, E., Dinan, C., Johnson, R. & Han, K.-H. 1997. Force-time dependent characteristics of dynamic and isometric muscle actions. *J Strength Cond Res*, 11, 269–72.

Haff, G. G. 2019. Strength – isometric and dynamic testing. *In*: Comfort, P., Jones, P. A. & McMahon, J. J. (eds). *Performance Assessment in Strength and Conditioning*. New York, NY: Routledge.

Haff, G. G., Carlock, J. M., Hartman, M. J., Kilgore, J. L., Kawamori, N., Jackson, J. R., Morris, R. T., Sands, W. A. & Stone, M. H. 2005. Force-time curve characteristics of dynamic and isometric muscle actions of elite women Olympic weightlifters. *J Strength Cond Res*, 19, 741–8.

Haff, G. G., Ruben, R. P., Lider, J., Twine, C. & Cormie, P. 2015. A comparison of methods for determining the rate of force development during isometric mid-thigh clean pulls. *J Strength Cond Res*, 29, 386–95.

Halperin, I., Williams, K. J., Martin, D. T. & Chapman, D. W. 2016. The effects of attentional focusing instructions on force production during the isometric midthigh pull. *J Strength Cond Res*, 30, 919–23.

Hori, N., Newton, R. U., Andrews, W. A., Kawamori, N., Mcguigan, M. R. & Nosaka, K. 2008. Does performance of hang power clean differentiate performance of jumping, sprinting, and changing of direction? *J Strength Cond Res*, 22, 412–8.

Hornsby, W., Gentles, J., Macdonald, C., Mizuguchi, S., Ramsey, M. & Stone, M. 2017. Maximum strength, rate of force development, jump height, and peak power alterations in weightlifters across five months of training. *Sports*, 5, 78.

Julio, U. F., Panissa, V. L. G. & Franchini, E. 2012. Prediction of one repetition maximum from the maximum number of repetitions with submaximal loads in recreationally strength-trained men. *Sci Sports*, 27, e69–76.

Lauersen, J. B., Andersen, T. E. & Andersen, L. B. 2018. Strength training as superior, dose-dependent and safe prevention of acute and overuse sports injuries: A systematic review, qualitative analysis and meta-analysis. *Br J Sports Med*, 52, 1557–65.

Lauersen, J. B., Bertelsen, D. M. & Andersen, L. B. 2014. The effectiveness of exercise interventions to prevent sports injuries: A systematic review and meta-analysis of randomised controlled trials. *Br J Sports Med*, 48, 871–7.

Maffiuletti, N. A., Aagaard, P., Blazevich, A. J., Folland, J., Tillin, N. & Duchateau, J. 2016. Rate of force development: Physiological and methodological considerations. *Eur J Appl Physiol*, 116, 1091–116.

Malone, S., Hughes, B., Doran, D. A., Collins, K. & Gabbett, T. J. 2019. Can the workload-injury relationship be moderated by improved strength, speed and repeated-sprint qualities? *J Sci Med Sport*, 22, 29–34.

Morales, J. & Sobonya, S. 1996. Use of submaximal repetition tests for predicting 1-RM strength in class athletes. *J Strength Cond Res*, 10, 186–9.

Nimphius, S. 2018. Re-evaluating what we "know" about female athletes in biomechanics research: Across the continuum from capacity to skill. *ISBS Proc Arch*, 36, 1059.

Nimphius, S. 2019. Exercise and sport science failing by design in understanding female athletes. *Int J Sports Physiol Perform*, 14, 1157–8.

Nimphius, S., Mcguigan, M. R. & Newton, R. U. 2010. Relationship between strength, power, speed, and change of direction performance of female softball players. *J Strength Cond Res*, 24, 885–95.

Nuzzo, J. L., Mcbride, J. M., Cormie, P. & Mccaulley, G. O. 2008. Relationship between countermovement jump performance and multijoint isometric and dynamic tests of strength. *J Strength Cond Res*, 22, 699–707.

Sayers, M. G. L., Schlaeppi, M., Hitz, M. & Lorenzetti, S. 2018. The impact of test loads on the accuracy of 1RM prediction using the load-velocity relationship. *BMC Sports Sci Med Rehabil*, 10, 9.

Seitz, L. B., Reyes, A., Tran, T. T., De Villarreal, E. S. & Haff, G. G. 2014. Increases in lower-body strength transfer positively to sprint performance: A systematic review with meta-analysis. *Sports Med*, 44, 1693–702.

Styles, W. J., Matthews, M. J. & Comfort, P. 2015. Effects of strength training on squat and sprint performance in soccer players. *J Strength Cond Res*, 30, 1534–9.

Suarez, D. G., Mizuguchi, S., Hornsby, W. G., Cunanan, A. J., Marsh, D. J. & Stone, M. H. 2019. Phase-specific changes in rate of force development and muscle morphology throughout a block periodized training cycle in weightlifters. *Sports*, 7, 129.

Suchomel, T. J., Nimphius, S. & Stone, M. H. 2016. The importance of muscular strength in athletic performance. *Sports Med*, 46, 1419–49.

Suchomel, T. J., Nimphius, S. & Stone, M. H. 2018. Scaling isometric mid-thigh pull maximum strength in division in athletes: Are we meeting the assumptions? *Sports Biomech*, 1–15.

Verhoeff, W. J., Millar, S. K., Oldham, A. R. H. & Cronin, J. 2020. Coaching the power clean: A constraints-led approach. *Strength Cond J*, 42, 16–25.

Wisloff, U., Castagna, C., Helgerud, J., Jones, R. & Hoff, J. 2004. Strong correlation of maximal squat strength with sprint performance and vertical jump height in elite soccer players. *Br J Sports Med*, 38, 285–8.

7 Muscular Power

John McMahon and Paul Comfort

Part 1: Background

Introduction

Power has been a cause of confusion within the scientific literature (Winter et al., 2016). This is partly because of power being used as a qualitative term to describe performance within sports or athletic tasks rather than as a true definition of mechanical power (Knudson, 2009). Consequently, several peer-reviewed articles about power have been published to promote a universal understanding of what power means from a mechanical point of view, particularly among the strength and conditioning community (Knudson, 2009; Winter et al., 2016), although the term is still commonly used incorrectly. In brief, power is defined as the rate of performing mechanical work. Mechanical work describes the distance over which force is applied. It is calculated as force multiplied by displacement. Displacement can be thought of as the distance and direction travelled between two points, with ascending vertical (and forward horizontal) displacement often prescribed a positive number and descending vertical (and backward horizontal) displacement often prescribed a negative number. It is important to note that we choose our two points of interest when calculating displacement. In the descent phase of a squat, for example, point A could be our centre of mass (COM) position when standing upright and point B could be our lowest COM position in the squat and this would be prescribed a negative value, such as −0.5 m. Mechanical work is greater if either a larger force has been applied over the same displacement or the same force has been applied over a larger displacement. In either of these two scenarios, power would be greater if the mechanical work was performed in a shorter time. Power can also be calculated as force multiplied by velocity, due to velocity equalling displacement divided by time (see equations later). The Système International (SI) unit for power is Watt (W). Despite force, displacement and velocity being "vector quantities" (i.e., having both a magnitude and direction), both mechanical work and power are "scalar quantities" (i.e., having a magnitude, but no direction) (Winter et al., 2016), although their numeric values are usually assigned a direction in line with the aforementioned convention in order to facilitate data interpretation. The two primary equations for calculating power are shown here:

$$Power = work \div time \tag{7.1}$$

DOI: 10.4324/9781003186762-7

Thus:

$$Power = (force \times displacement) \div time$$

Thus:

$$Power = force \times (displacement \div time)$$

Thus:

$$Power = force \times velocity \qquad\qquad (7.2)$$

Why Measure Power?

Strength and conditioning researchers and practitioners might be interested in measuring power because it describes the ability to generate a high output (work) in a short time which has been highlighted as a performance-determining factor for many high-level athletes (Baker and Nance, 1999; Cormie et al., 2011; Haff and Nimphius, 2012). This is because the time available to most athletes for producing force, and therefore velocity and power, when they are performing their sport, is limited. Thus, in sports, whereby the requirement for attaining a high velocity in the associated underpinning athletic actions but over a short time is paramount, the ability to produce high power outputs, and therefore assess this ability, is useful. However, because a greater power output is attained by producing either (1) a larger amount of work over the same time, (2) the same amount of work over a shorter time, or (3) a larger amount of work over a shorter time (the ideal scenario), it can be more illuminating for the strength and conditioning coach to deconstruct power output into its composite parts (including the involved force and displacement and the phases [where applicable] within the test for which power is calculated).

Part 2: Assessing Power

Assessments of power output within the field of strength and conditioning generally involves a vertical jump test. Thus, this primary "power assessment" type alone will be discussed in detail within this section, although the readers should be aware that power can be assessed during many other tasks, such as cycling [typically on an ergometer] and weightlifting derivatives.

Vertical Jump Tests

Firstly, vertical *jump height is not a measure of power*, despite it often being suggested to describe leg power during a variety of jump tests. The most common vertical jump test conducted with athletes is the countermovement jump. While it is true that power can be measured during vertical jump tests, and power will usually be greatest for unloaded (i.e., just bodyweight) versus externally loaded vertical jumps, a higher jump is not always a consequence of higher power output. This can be explained due to jump height being underpinned by a greater mechanical work but not the rate with which it is produced. Thus, it is true to say that when a higher jump has been achieved, that greater mechanical work relative to body mass must have been done during the propulsion (i.e., concentric) phase (i.e., when extending hips, knees, and ankles from the lowest COM position during the jump through to the instant of leaving the ground). However, the power output is only guaranteed to have been greater if the higher jump was achieved with the same or a shorter propulsion phase time (refer back to Equation 7.1). See examples of this notion in Part 3, as part of case studies 1 and 2. The reason for moderate-to-large correlations between both peak and mean propulsion power and countermovement jump height ($r = 0.54$–0.90) is suggested to be due the large correlations between the velocity at peak power (during the propulsion phase) and countermovement jump height (Linthorne, 2021). In other words, relationships between propulsion power and countermovement jump height are artificially inflated due to the almost perfect relation ($r = 0.83$–0.94) between the corresponding propulsion velocity at peak power and countermovement jump height (Linthorne, 2021). To facilitate visualization for the reader, the point within which propulsion peak power occurs during the countermovement jump is shown in Figure 7.1. The reason that propulsion velocity at peak power and countermovement jump height are so highly correlated is due to the velocity at take-off, which will be greater if the mean propulsion velocity and therefore the propulsion velocity at peak power are greater, dictating vertical jump height (Mcbride et al., 2010; Kirby et al., 2011). The reason that velocity at take-off dictates vertical jump height can be explained by both

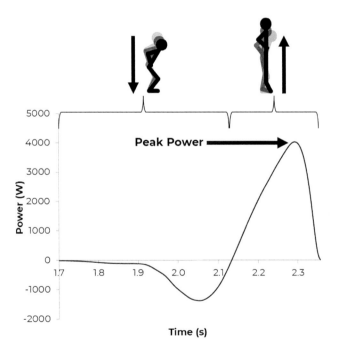

Figure 7.1 An illustration of where peak power occurs during the countermovement jump. The portion of the power-time curve underneath the braces associated with the downward and upward arrows denotes the countermovement (negative power values) and propulsion (positive power values) phases, respectively.

the equation for one-dimensional motion and the conservation of mechanical energy principle (Linthorne, 2001). Both approaches result in the same simplified formula for calculating jump height from take-off velocity shown here:

$$\frac{v^2}{2g} = h \tag{7.3}$$

Where v is vertical take-off velocity, g is gravitational acceleration and h is jump height.

Power can be directly measured if vertical jump tests are performed on a force plate system, which is becoming increasingly common in sport owing to affordable, but valid, systems being widely available (Peterson Silveira et al., 2016; Lake et al., 2018). Even though equations exist that enable the prediction of power from jump height and body mass (Güçlüöver and Gülü, 2020), which may be pertinent when a force plate is not used to assess vertical jump performance, their efficacy in respect to categorizing and ranking athletes' power output has been challenged (Ache-Dias et al., 2016) and if used, used with caution. Additionally, linear position transducers have also been used as a standalone device to measure power applied to either a portion of the body (usually the hips to reflect the approximate whole-body COM location) or a barbell. However, it has been reported that these methods cannot be used interchangeably for measuring power output during bodyweight only and externally loaded vertical jumps (Mundy et al., 2016). As described in Chapter 4, the strength and conditioning coach may wish to determine the concurrent validity of power assessment devices themselves, especially if they are using a system which has not been validated in a peer-reviewed study.

Force Plates

Force plates measure the ground reaction force [when placed on the ground, otherwise this may be referred to as the normal reaction force] which is the mirror image (equal in magnitude but opposite in direction) of the force that the athlete imparts onto them during a given task. The ground reaction force represents the forces applied from the force plate back to the athlete's whole-body COM. Thus, it does not inform us of which joints, segments, or muscles are predominantly responsibly for producing the involved force(s). In the case of the vertical jump, specifically the countermovement jump, the vertical component of the ground reaction force is usually collected at 1000 Hz (Owen et al., 2014) for *individual repetitions* over a 5-second period (thus leading to 5000 individual samples of force per trial). A representative ground reaction force-time series for the countermovement jump is presented in Figure 7.2.

To be able to calculate power accurately from the recorded ground reaction force, there are several steps that the strength and conditioning coach (the assumed test conductor) is responsible for. Firstly, the force plate must firstly be placed on *firm and level ground, zeroed* before the athlete steps onto it, and set to a minimum of *1000 Hz, if possible* (but ideally no less than 500 Hz). Then, the athlete must *remain still and upright for at least one second* prior to performing the jump (Owen et al., 2014), but while the data are being recorded, to allow post-measurement of body weight and the initial COM position to be set to zero, respectively. It is advised that the athletes place *their hands on their hips* prior to the jump trial being recorded via the force plate and

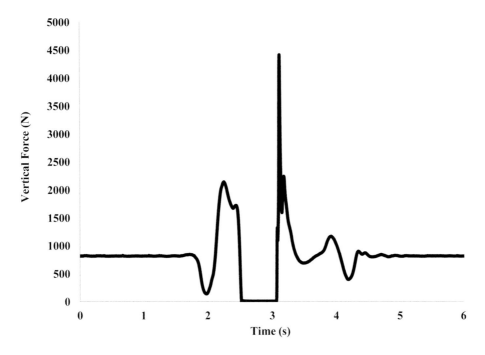

Figure 7.2 A representative countermovement jump force-time curve collected via a force plate.

keep them there throughout the entire trial. This is to standardise the test to limit both within- and between-athlete variation in arm swing technique (Markovic et al., 2004) and therefore isolate the lower body contribution to the jump. Remember, the ground reaction force-time series will not inform us of which joints, segments, or muscles produced the force, so constraining the upper limb contribution to the task will help us better hone in on this principally lower body activity. Finally, it is essential that all athletes are *verbally instructed* on how to perform the vertical jump test in the same manner (Sánchez-Sixto et al., in press). For most vertical jump tests, the athletes will likely be cued to jump as fast (meaning to leave the ground quickly) and high as possible, rather than just to focus on maximising jump height, which should elicit a larger power output (see subsequent sections for a detailed discussion of this).

The strength and conditioning coach is unlikely to be responsible for analysing the ground reaction force data obtained for each vertical jump trial. Instead, commercial force plate software is likely to be utilized for this purpose, meaning there is a reliance on the provider for ensuring accuracy in the power measurement. An explanation of the typical process of calculating power from the vertical jump ground reaction force-time series is provided here, but the author encourages the strength and conditioning coach to request the data analysis methods employed by their commercial force plate software provider, as they tend to yield slightly different results (Merrigan et al., 2022).

When jumping vertically, the athletes must overcome their bodyweight, and so the resultant force (commonly referred to as the net force) acting on the athletes' COM is required when exploring the influence of applied force on COM motion, which is needed to calculate power (Linthorne, 2001). The net force acting on the athletes'

COM is calculated by subtracting their bodyweight (usually calculated as the mean force over at least a one-second period where the athlete remained upright and still) from the entire vertical ground reaction force-time series. Based on known associations between mechanical variables, that are governed by Newton's laws of motion, it is possible to obtain other kinetic and kinematic variables, including power, from the original (or filtered) ground reaction force-time series. The underpinning mathematical process applied to the ground reaction force-time series is called *numerical integration* and the overarching process is often referred to as forward dynamics. The simplest way of calculating power is to apply Equation 7.2, but do to so, it is a requirement to first calculate the COM velocity. For the velocity-time series for a vertical jump trial to be obtained, the acceleration-time series must first be calculated. This is achieved by dividing the net ground reaction force-time series by the athlete's body mass (with body mass usually calculated by dividing body weight by an assumed constant gravitational acceleration of 9.81 m/s^2) on a sample-by-sample basis (for every 0.001 s sample when the sample rate is set to 1000 Hz). The acceleration-time series is then numerically integrated with respect to time using the trapezoid rule to give the velocity-time series. The power-time series for the vertical jump can then be calculated by multiplying the ground reaction force by velocity on a sample-by-sample basis.

Equation 7.1 for calculating power can also be applied to force plate assessments of vertical jumping but further steps are required. Specifically, to calculate work, the displacement-time series is first obtained by numerically integrating the velocity-time series, again using the trapezoid rule. This is often referred to as numerical double integration of the ground reaction force-time series. Numerical double integration is very reliant upon accurate body mass determination (Vanrenterghem et al., 2001) which is another reason why it is very important for the athletes to remain motionless for at least one second prior to performing the jump. Once the displacement-time series has been calculated, the work done on the athlete's COM can be calculated by multiplying ground reaction force by displacement on a sample-by-sample basis.

It is important to note that power is usually reported as the mean or peak value over a specific vertical jump phase of interest. Usually, power (whether mean or peak) is reported solely for the propulsion phase (i.e., when extending hips, knees, and ankles from the lowest COM position during the jump through to the instant of leaving the ground). The power attained in the propulsion phase will be larger than in any other phase of the jump because this is the phase within which the highest velocity is obtained (Linthorne, 2021). The peak propulsion power represents the single highest instantaneous power value obtained within this phase, whereas the mean propulsion power represents the average power applied over the entirety of this phase. However, the average power is somewhat influenced by the thresholds utilized by the software provider to identify the onset and end of the propulsion phase (Merrigan et al., 2022). Finally, it is typical for strength and conditioning coaches to wish to report the mean and/or peak propulsion power values relative to each athlete's body mass which is achieved by simply dividing each power variant by body mass (either themselves or this will be done by the software used). Sometimes, power may be the only variable reported following a vertical jump test on a force plate or perhaps it will be reported alongside the vertical jump height. In either case, this provides a narrow view of the vertical jump performance and makes it impossible to know how the power was achieved by athlete and/or how it changed since the last time they were tested. To better understand power, it would be prudent for the strength and conditioning coach to deconstruct power output into its composite parts, as mentioned earlier and which is discussed as part of the practical examples provided in Part 3.

Part 3: Practical Examples

Case Study 1: Baseline Power Testing

Two senior male professional rugby league players (both forwards) performed three maximal effort countermovement jumps as part of their club's early pre-season testing programme using a portable dual force plate system. Athlete 1 had a body mass of 112 kg and athlete 2 had a body mass of 95 kg.

Both peak and mean propulsion power were automatically calculated by the commercial software used and expressed both in absolute terms (W) and relative to each athlete's body mass (W/kg). The absolute and relative peak and mean propulsion power values are presented in Table 7.1 along with some other countermovement jump variables that were also calculated from the ground reaction force-time series (all recorded as the average of the three countermovement jump trials). The position average and SD values for each metric are also presented (Table 7.1).

The first thing to note is that absolute peak propulsion power is larger for athlete 1 but the relative peak propulsion power is larger for athlete 2, as is the mean propulsion power when expressed both in absolute and relative terms (Table 7.1). These differences highlight that the precise power "variant" selected can potentially alter the strength and conditioning coach's test interpretation and lead to different training recommendations. With the additional variables presented in Table 7.1, the strength and conditioning coach can determine how the power outputs were achieved by each athlete. For example, athlete 2 achieved a higher absolute mean propulsion power despite performing less propulsion work (comprised of a higher mean propulsion force applied over a lower propulsion displacement) due to their propulsion time being much lower. The lower propulsion time is likely due in part to the lower propulsion displacement (McMahon et al., 2022a). The jump height was larger for

Table 7.1 Select countermovement jump variables derived from a force plate for two senior male professional rugby league players (both forwards) and the position average (Avg.) and standard deviation (SD) values.

	Absolute Peak Power (W)	Absolute Mean Power (W)	Absolute Mean Force (N)	Propulsion Displacement (m)	Propulsion Time (s)
Athlete 1	6080	2932	2019	0.50	0.319
Athlete 2	5276	3150	2114	0.36	0.216
Position Avg.	5201	2925	2012	0.43	0.266
Position SD	707	417	202	0.06	0.036

	Relative Peak Power (W/kg)	Relative Mean Power (W/kg)	Relative Mean Force (N/kg)	Propulsion Work (J)	Jump Height (m)
Athlete 1	54.4	26.2	18.1	385	0.35
Athlete 2	55.7	33.3	22.3	350	0.37
Position Avg.	50.3	28.3	19.5	347	0.34
Position SD	6.8	4.0	2.0	11	0.04

athlete 2 despite their propulsion work being lower due to them being lighter. Athlete 2's lighter body mass also likely contributed to them being able to perform the countermovement jump with a much shorter propulsion time, as illustrated by the steeper power-time series gradient in Figure 7.3. These results highlight the benefit of reporting supplementary variables to power output in order to facilitate the strength and conditioning coach's understanding of how it was attained by each athlete.

In addition to comparing the athlete's power data to the average (mean) obtained by athletes from the same position group (i.e., forwards) within their squad, the data may

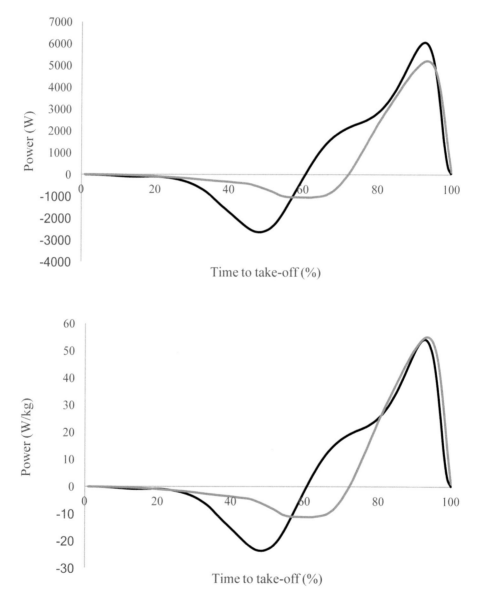

Figure 7.3 The countermovement jump power-time curves (absolute power shown in top graph and relative power shown in bottom graph) of two senior male professional rugby league players (both forwards; athlete 1 = black line; athlete 2 = grey line).

also be compared to published normative data provided that a similar test protocol was adhered to. In this case study example, the test protocol and data analyses procedures were very similar to a published study in which percentiles for the countermovement jump mean and peak propulsion power (relative to body mass) attained by professional male rugby league players were reported (McMahon et al., 2022b). Based on this study, athlete 1 would be placed in the 70–75th percentile for relative peak propulsion power but the 20–25th percentile for relative mean propulsion power, whereas athlete 2 would be placed in the 80–85th percentile for relative peak propulsion power and the 85–90th percentile for relative mean propulsion power (McMahon et al., 2022b). Thus, power development would likely not be a primary forthcoming training priority for athlete 2, but possibly would be for athlete 1. It is important to note that other physical qualities that are deemed to be important for the athletes' position within their sport, such as maximal strength (see Chapter 6), maximal short-distance speed (see Chapter 11), and change of direction ability (see Chapter 12), should also be considered alongside their power output for a more informed training programme.

Case Study 2: Monitoring Power Changes

A senior female professional soccer player performed three maximal effort counter-movement jumps as part of her club's early pre-season testing programme and then again fifteen weeks later, after completing a strength followed by a power-focussed training programme for the lower body. On both occasions, the athlete was tested using a portable dual force plate system. The athlete's body mass was 70 kg at the start of the training programme (at baseline testing) and 63 kg at the end of the training programme (at post-testing).

Both peak and mean propulsion power were automatically calculated on each test occasion by the commercial software used and expressed both in absolute terms (W) and relative to the athlete's body mass (W/kg). The absolute and relative peak and mean propulsion power values are presented in Table 7.2 along with some other countermovement jump variables that were also calculated from the ground reaction force-time series both before and after the strength training programme was completed (all recorded as the average of the three countermovement jump trials).

Table 7.2 Select countermovement jump variables derived from a force plate for a senior female professional soccer player before and after a fifteen-week-long power-focussed training programme.

	Absolute Peak Power (W)	*Absolute Mean Power (W)*	*Absolute Mean Force (N)*	*Propulsion Displacement (m)*	*Propulsion Time (s)*
Pre-test	3069	1763	2019	0.46	0.300
Post-test	2712	1579	2114	0.39	0.263
Change (units)	−357	−184	95	−0.07	−0.037
Change (%)	−11.6	−10.4	4.7	−16.1	−12.3

	Relative Peak Power (W/kg)	*Relative Mean Power (W/kg)*	*Relative Mean Force (N/kg)*	*Propulsion Work (J)*	*Jump Height (m)*
Pre-test	43.8	25.2	28.8	217	0.31
Post-test	42.8	24.9	33.3	179	0.28
Change (units)	−1.0	−0.3	4.5	−38	−0.03
Change (%)	−2.4	−1.0	15.7	−17.5	−9.7

The first thing to note is that power output (all variants) reduced following the fifteen-week training programme. However, the absolute peak and mean propulsion power seen much larger reductions that the relative values due to the athlete losing 7 kg of body mass. Additionally, the post-test reductions in relative peak (2.4%) and mean (1%) propulsion power are so small (also see Figure 7.4) that they are likely less than the measurement error (Mercer et al., 2021) and so may be interpreted

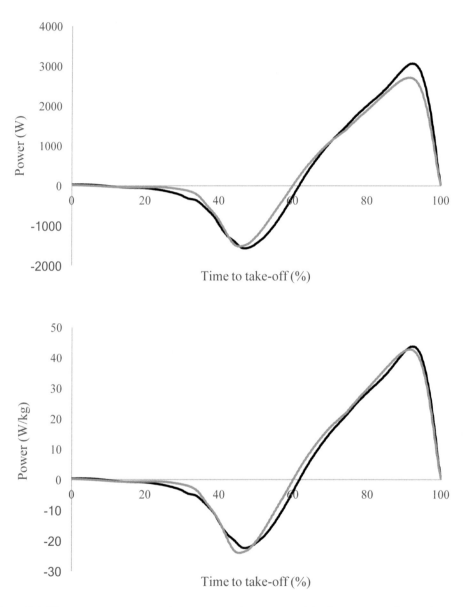

Figure 7.4 The countermovement jump power-time curves (absolute power shown in top graph and relative power shown in bottom graph) for a senior female professional soccer player before (black line) and after (grey line) a 15-week-long power-focussed training programme.

as not changing compared with the pre-test values. At face value, the strength and conditioning coach may conclude that the fifteen-week training programme had no effect on the athlete's relative power output. Furthermore, the accompanying large post-test reduction in jump height (a marker of reduced velocity) may be viewed as a negative outcome of the training programme. But the additional variables reported in Table 7.2 help contextualise the reasons for no change and a reduction in power output and jump height, respectively. For example, in the post-test, the athlete performed the propulsion phase of the jump with a larger relative mean force applied over a shorter displacement and, therefore, a reduced time. Essentially, the athlete had changed their jump strategy in the post-test, opting for a stiffer leg approach (reduced peak ankle, knee, and hip flexion) with the resulting heightened force not outweighing the reduced displacement and time during propulsion, which equalized the pre-test power output (less work but produced in less time) but reduced jump height (less work and net impulse [mean force × time]). Thus, it is not accurate to say that the athlete maintained (power output) or reduced (jump height) their jump performance following the training intervention, but rather it is more complex than that. Also, these results highlight that jump height should not be used as a surrogate for power. Should the athlete adopt the same jump strategy (i.e., propulsion displacement and time) and maintain body mass after a further period of training, the only way in which their power output and jump height will increase is if they are able to apply a larger propulsion force.

Laboratory Task: How "Powerful" Are You?

As explained in the two case studies presented earlier, power output is very dependent on jump strategy (i.e., how the athlete performs the jump with regards to COM displacement and movement duration) and body mass, which is why it is important to report more than just power, and, indeed, jump height, following a vertical jump assessment performed on a force plate. The authors encourage you to experiment with various jump strategies to further illustrate their influence on power output by completing the laboratory task outlined later.

Task Instructions

Complete three maximal effort countermovement jumps to various depths on a force plate, if possible. Specially, perform one countermovement jump to your preferred depth, one shallower than preferred (i.e., less ankle, knee, and hip flexion during countermovement phase of the jump [shallower squat]) and one to a deeper than preferred (i.e., more ankle, knee, and hip flexion during countermovement phase of the jump [deeper squat]). Acquire the force data per the manufacturer's guidelines, adhering to the recommended data collection steps described in Part 2, where possible. What do you notice about your propulsion power output, whether peak or mean? According to previous work, it is anticipated that power output will be greatest for the shallower (i.e., stiffer) and lowest for the deeper (i.e., more compliant) jump trials, when compared with the preferred trial (McMahon et al., 2016).

If you do not have access to a force plate, the authors recommend that you complete the same task outlined earlier but with an alternative device that is available to you (e.g., phone application, jump mat, etc.). Instead of focussing on power this time, as these alternative devices likely do not provide power metrics, focus on jump height. What do you notice about your jump height? According to previous work, it is anticipated jump height will be greatest for the deeper (i.e., more compliant) and lowest for the shallower (i.e., stiffer) jump trials, when compared with the preferred trial (McMahon et al., 2016).

This laboratory task should help emphasize the importance of consistent verbal cueing of athletes when conducting vertical jump tests as well as the limitations of reporting more than just power output and jump height when conducting such tests with athletes. This task can also be performed after a change in body mass has occurred (e.g., after a period of physical training has taken place) and with the inclusion of arm swing to facilitate the reader's understanding of the interplay between these factors and both power output and jump height.

Summary

It is undoubtedly important for most athletes to be able to generate high power outputs to be successful in their respective sport. How the strength and conditioning coach assesses power should be considered carefully, however, with particular attention paid to test standardization and complimentary metrics. Understanding how a certain power output was attained for different athletes and/or how it changed or remained the same after a period of training or competition is essential to better direct athletes' training programmes.

References

Ache-Dias, J., Dal Pupo, J., Gheller, R. G., Külkamp, W. & Moro, A. R. P. 2016. Power output prediction from jump height and body mass does not appropriately categorize or rank athletes. *J Strength Cond Res*, 30, 818–24.

Baker, D. & Nance, S. 1999. The relation between strength and power in professional Rugby league players. *J Strength Cond Res*, 13, 224–9.

Cormie, P., Mcguigan, M. R. & Newton, R. U. 2011. Developing maximal neuromuscular power: Part 1–biological basis of maximal power production. *Sports Med*, 41, 17–38.

Güçlüöver, A. & Gülü, M. 2020. Developing a new muscle power prediction equation through vertical jump power output in adolescent women. *Medicine*, 99, e20882.

Haff, G. G. & Nimphius, S. 2012. Training principles for power. *Strength Cond J*, 34, 2–12.

Kirby, T. J., Mcbride, J. M., Haines, T. L. & Dayne, A. M. 2011. Relative net vertical impulse determines jumping performance. *J Appl Biomech*, 27, 207–14.

Knudson, D. V. 2009. Correcting the use of the term "Power" in the strength and conditioning literature. *J Strength Cond Res*, 23, 1902–8.

Lake, J., Mundy, P., Comfort, P., McMahon, J. J., Suchomel, T. J. & Carden, P. 2018. Concurrent validity of a portable force plate using vertical jump force-time characteristics. *J Appl Biomech*, 34, 410–3.

Linthorne, N. P. 2001. Analysis of standing vertical jumps using a force platform. *Am J Phys*, 69, 1198–204.

Linthorne, N. P. 2021. The correlation between jump height and mechanical power in a countermovement jump is artificially inflated. *Sports Biomech*, 20, 3–21.

Markovic, G., Dizdar, D., Jukic, I. & Cardinale, M. 2004. Reliability and factorial validity of squat and countermovement jump tests. *J Strength Cond Res*, 18, 551–5.

Mcbride, J. M., Kirby, T. J., Haines, T. L. & Skinner, J. 2010. Relationship between relative net vertical impulse and jump height in jump squats performed to various squat depths and with various loads. *Int J Sports Physiol Perform*, 5, 484–96.

McMahon, J. J., Jones, P. A. & Comfort, P. 2022a. Comparison of countermovement jump-derived reactive strength index modified and underpinning force-time variables between super league and championship rugby league players. *J Strength Cond Res*, 36, 226–31.

McMahon, J. J., Lake, J. P., Dos' Santos, T., Jones, P., Thomasson, M. & Comfort, P. 2022b. Countermovement jump standards in rugby league: What is a 'good' performance? *J Strength Cond Res*, 36, 1691–8.

McMahon, J. J., Ripley, N. J. & Rej, S. J. 2016. Effect of modulating eccentric leg stiffness on concentric force-velocity characteristics demonstrated in the countermovement jump. *J Sports Sci*, 34, S19.

Mercer, R. A. J., Russell, J. L., Mcguigan, L. C., Coutts, A. J., Strack, D. S. & Mclean, B. D. 2021. Finding the signal in the noise—Interday reliability and seasonal sensitivity of 84 countermovement jump variables in professional basketball players. *J Strength Cond Res*, published ahead-of-print.

Merrigan, J. J., Stone, J. D., Galster, S. M. & Hagen, J. A. 2022. Analyzing force-time curves: Comparison of commercially available automated software and custom MATLAB analyses. *J Strength Cond Res*, 36(9), 2387–2402, published ahead-of-print. 10.1519/JSC.0000000000004275.

Mundy, P. D., Lake, J. P., Carden, P. J. C., Smith, N. A. & Lauder, M. A. 2016. Agreement between the force platform method and the combined method measurements of power output during the loaded countermovement jump. *Sports Biom*, 15, 23–35.

Owen, N. J., Watkins, J., Kilduff, L. P., Bevan, H. R. & Bennett, M. A. 2014. Development of a criterion method to determine peak mechanical power output in a countermovement jump. *J Strength Cond Res*, 28, 1552–8.

Peterson Silveira, R., Stergiou, P., Carpes, F. P., Castro, F. A. D. S., Katz, L. & Stefanyshyn, D. J. 2016. Validity of a portable force platform for assessing biomechanical parameters in three different tasks. *Sports Biom*, 16, 177–86.

Sánchez-Sixto, A., McMahon, J. J. & Floría, P. In press. Verbal instructions affect reactive strength index modified and time-series waveforms in basketball players. *Sports Biom*.

Vanrenterghem, J., De Clercq, D. & Cleven, P. V. 2001. Necessary precautions in measuring correct vertical jumping height by means of force plate measurements. *Ergonomics*, 44, 814–8.

Winter, E. M., Abt, G., Brookes, F. B. C., Challis, J. H., Fowler, N. E., Knudson, D. V., Knuttgen, H. G., Kraemer, W. J., Lane, A. M., Mechelen, W. V., Morton, R. H., Newton, R. U., Williams, C. & Yeadon, M. R. 2016. Misuse of "Power" and other mechanical terms in sport and exercise science research. *J Strength Cond Res*, 30, 292–300.

8 Muscular Endurance

Paul Comfort and John McMahon

Part 1: Introduction

Muscular endurance tends to be assessed for a variety of reasons, with the most obvious being to determine the work capacity of a muscle group (i.e., single joint task) or series of muscles (i.e., multi-joint task). Muscular endurance protocols are also sometimes used to predict maximal strength or to evaluate muscular characteristics in individuals who may not be competent in performing exercises with maximal or near maximal loads, and in some cases, where a maximal load test is not feasible (e.g., plank and abdominal crunch). Due to the higher reliability and lower measurement error associated with maximal strength testing, where possible, the assessment of maximal strength would be preferential to the assessment of muscular endurance. However, muscular endurance tests are commonly used in fitness batteries for children and adolescents (Castro-Piñero et al., 2010; Lubans et al., 2011), in health-related settings and research (Cantell et al., 2008; Bianco et al., 2015) and in certain physically demanding occupations (e.g., police and military) (Barringer et al., 2019; Lockie et al., 2020), as they are easy to perform on mass with minimal equipment. However, appropriate familiarization with the tasks is required as a learning effect and systematic bias has been noted in some studies (Lubans et al., 2011).

Interestingly, while these tests are commonly viewed as having a lower risk of injury than a one repetition maximum (1 RM), as fatigue ensues during a muscular endurance test technique is likely to progressively deteriorate, and therefore should be continually and closely monitored. If technique becomes an issue and the correct posture (e.g., loss of neutral spine) or movement pattern is not being maintained (e.g., increased hip flexion and reduced knee flexion during a deadlift or squat) the task should be terminated. Technique issues can also be observed during isometric assessments, usually as a loss of spinal alignment due to fatigue of the abdominal muscles, in which case the task should be stopped.

Interestingly, performing the maximum number of repetitions over a specific duration (e.g., the maximum number of repetitions in one minute) has been questioned as an appropriate method of evaluating endurance, due to movement speed and therefore muscular power being a contributing factor (Quinney et al., 1984; Sparling et al., 1997). As such, the efficacy and validity of any version of endurance tests which includes a timed component should be questioned.

DOI: 10.4324/9781003186762-8

Part 2: Muscular Endurance Assessments

Push-Up Tests

Numerous different protocols have been employed for the push-up test, including the 90° push-up (e.g., where the range of motion is determined by flexing the elbows to 90° and returning to full extension) (McManis et al., 2000; Lubans et al., 2011; Hashim et al., 2018) and the full push-up where the chest is lowered to a specific height (e.g., a rolled-up towel, or a water bottle led flat; Lockie et al. (2020), or until the chest touches the floor (Pate et al., 1993; Ojeda et al., 2020). The test has also been modified to accommodate individuals who lack the strength to perform the push-up supported on their hands and toes, by performing it on an incline with the hands on a bench of a standardized height (e.g., 13 inches), or the bent knee push-up, where the individual is supported on their hands and knees (commonly adopted when testing females (Haugen et al., 2013)), reducing the moment arm and the load through the upper body (Baumgartner et al., 2002; Wood and Baumgartner, 2004; Hashim et al., 2018). While each of these tests appears to be reliable (McManis et al., 2000; Baumgartner et al., 2002; Wood and Baumgartner, 2004; Lubans et al., 2011; Hashim et al., 2018; Ojeda et al., 2020), they cannot be used interchangeably, due to the differences in range of motion and load that the upper body is subjected to. As such, comparison between published data can only be completed if the same protocol has been used, and testing protocols are standardized for longitudinal monitoring of athletic development, to ensure that appropriate conclusions are drawn.

Testing Protocol

The athlete should be positioned with only their toes and hands in contact with the floor, with their hands slightly wider than shoulder width, resulting in ~45° angle between the trunk and the humerus. They should then flex their elbows to lower their chest to the floor and then return back to the start position with their arms fully extended (Figure 8.1). To standardize the cadence of the repetition a metronome set at 40 beats per minute can be used to ensure that one repetition is performed every 3 seconds (Lubans et al., 2011). During the movement the athlete should keep their body in a straight line, maintaining a neutral spinal posture, with a rigid torso and no movement through the hips. If the individual is not strong enough to perform the push-up in this manner, they should perform them on their knees (Figure 8.2). The total number of repetitions completed with good techniques is the final score. Normative data for adults are presented in Table 8.1, with data for adolescents in Table 8.2.

Pull-Up Test

This test should be implemented with caution in children and adolescents as for many individuals, this is a strength test rather than endurance test (based on the low number of repetitions that many individuals can perform). In fact, Woods et al. (1992) suggested that the pull-up test is not an appropriate or valid test of muscular endurance in adolescents as many individuals are not strong enough to perform a single full repetition. For example, Castro-Piñero et al. (2010) reported, in a systematic review,

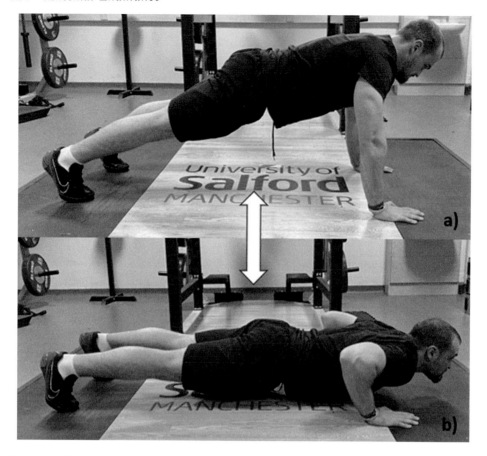

Figure 8.1 Push-up test sequence, (a) represents the start and finish position of a repetition, and (b) represents the mid-point of the repetition.

that 85% of girls and 60% of boys were not able to complete a single repetition during the pull-up test. As such, some individuals opt for the 90° bent arm hang test (a test of isometric endurance). However, it has been reported that in adolescents, 39% of girls and 28% of boys cannot hold the isometric position, therefore questioning the validity of this test in adolescents (Castro-Piñero et al., 2010). Some adults are also not able to perform the test as an assessment of muscular endurance, with 81% of female and 8% of male law enforcement personnel, unable to perform more than two repetitions (Lockie et al., 2020). In contrast, in athletic adult populations, the pull-up endurance test has been reported to be highly reliable (intraclass correlation coefficient [ICC] ≥ 0.90) when following a standardized testing protocol (Vanderburgh and Edmonds, 1997; Sanchez-Moreno et al., 2016). For more information about reliability statistics, including the ICC, see Chapter 4.

Testing Protocol

The standardized protocol should consist of the individual taking a shoulder-width pronated grip on a pull-up bar. They should then hang with minimal movement

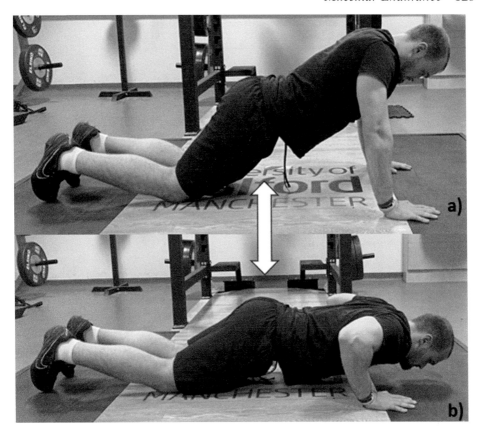

Figure 8.2 Modified push-up test sequence, (a) represents the start and finish position of a repetition, and (b) represents the mid-point of the repetition.

of the body and the arms fully extended, from there they should flex the elbows and pull the body up towards the bar (with no swinging or kicking of the legs, and no "kipping" motion) until the chin is above the bar (larynx level with the bar). The individual should then lower their body in a controlled manner until the arms are fully extended and then pause for 2 seconds until the tester instructs them to

Table 8.1 Percentiles for push-up performance.

Percentile	Repetitions
90–100	≥59
80–89	51–58
40–79	50
30–39	43–49
20–29	38–42
10–19	31–37
0–9	≤30

Data from Lockie et al. (2020).

Note: based on the maximum repetitions in 120 seconds.

Table 8.2 Percentiles for 90° push-up performance for adolescents.

Sex	Female			Male		
Age	13	14	15	13	14	15
Percentile			Repetitions			
90	35	42	50	30	40	48
75	30	33	40	24	31	40
50	21	25	30	17	22	30
25	18	18	21	10	16	21
10	9	11	15	5	10	13

Males performed push-ups on hands and toes, while females performed push-ups on hands and knees.

Data from Haugen et al. (2013).

perform the next repetition (Figure 8.3) in line with previous recommendations (Vanderburgh and Edmonds, 1997; Sanchez-Moreno et al., 2016). The maximum number of repetitions performed through a full range of motion should be taken as the athlete's score, with the final partial range of motion repetition excluded. Normative data, including percentiles, is provided in Table 8.3, based on the findings of Lockie et al. (2020).

Beckham et al. (2018) recently developed an equation to predict the maximum number of repetitions that can be performed, based on the mean concentric velocity

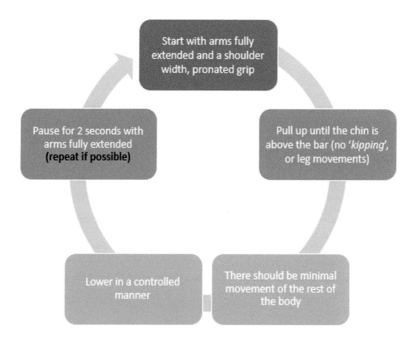

Figure 8.3 Standardized protocol for the pull-up endurance test.

Table 8.3 Percentiles for pull-up performance.

Percentile	Repetitions
90–100	≥21
80–89	16–20
70–79	13–15
60–69	11–12
50–59	10
40–49	8–9
30–39	6–7
20–29	3–5
13–19	1–2
0–12	0

Data from Lockie et al. (2020).

of the first repetition of the pull-up, where x is the mean concentric velocity and y is the maximum number of repetitions:

Female equation: $y = -4.062 + 19.381x$

Male equation: $y = -6.913 + 25.938x$

Prior to performing a maximal velocity pull-up, two warm-up sets of 5 repetitions using 50% body mass, one set of 3 repetitions using 75% body mass, and one single repetition at 100% body mass were performed on an assisted pull-up machine, with 90–120 seconds rest between sets. This was then followed by the one maximal velocity repetition, which is used to predict the maximum number of receptions (Beckham et al., 2018). It is worth noting that the velocity was evaluated using the GymAware PowerTool and that the mean concentric velocity may differ between devices if an alternative velocity assessment device is used (Fernandes et al., 2021; Weakley et al., 2021). In addition, if a linear position transducer is being used, it is essential that the device is appropriately placed and attached to the athlete to ensure that the chord is vertical, with minimal horizontal displacement throughout the exercise, to prevent the associated velocity from being inflated.

Curl-Up Test

The cadence (20 repetitions per minute) curl-up test has been shown to be reliable across ages and sexes (between session intraclass correlation coefficient [ICC] ≥ 0.70) (Plowman, 2013) and may be safer than the maximal effort timed curl-up tests (e.g., maximal repetitions performed in one minute), as technique is maintained better when performed at a steady cadence (Sparling et al., 1997; Plowman, 2013). In addition, as mentioned earlier, during a times test, muscular power is a contributing factor (Quinney et al., 1984; Sparling et al., 1997), potentially limiting the validity of the test.

Testing Protocol

The standardized posture (for the cadence curl-up test) is to lie supine on the floor with the calves resting on a box and the feet. The height of the box should permit the shins to be parallel to the floor and the knees flexed to 90°. Arms should be folded across the chest and shoulders in contact with the floor at the start of each repetition. The athlete should curl up and down in time with the beat of a metronome set at 40 bpm, with the elbows touching mid-thigh at the mid-point of each repetition (Figure 8.4). Performance is based on the maximal number of repetitions performed through the full range of motion at the desired cadence. Sparling et al. (1997) also reported that rectus femoris involvement is reduced when the feet are not anchored, which may be a better approach to determining the muscular endurance of the abdominal musculature.

In contrast, Sparling et al. (1997) evaluated curl-up test performance in college students, with the test performed for a maximum of three minutes (or until a successful repetition could not be completed) at a cadence of 25 repetitions per minute, to keep

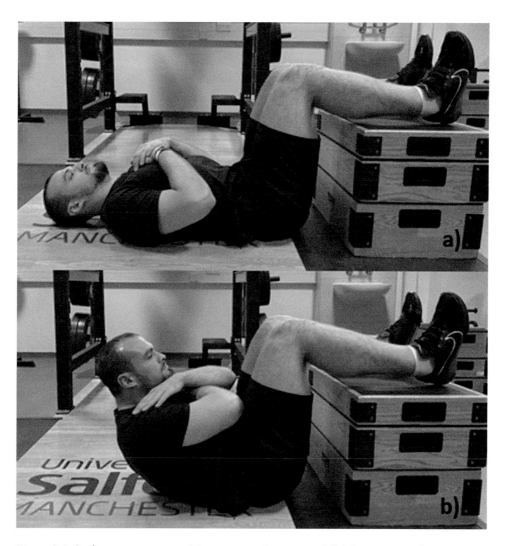

Figure 8.4 Curl-up test sequence, (a) represents the start and finish positions of a repetition, (b) represents the mid-point of the repetition.

it time-efficient, also reporting high between session reliability (ICC = 0.92). While it is recommended that the protocol described by Plowman (2013) is used, practitioners should be mindful of the fact that numerous variations of the curl-up protocol are used, which include different leg positions (e.g., feet on the floor at 90°) and different cadences, including the maximal number of repetitions performed in a given time, all of which affect the reliability and generalizability of the results. As such, when comparing athletes' performances to published "normative" values or benchmarks, it is essential that comparisons are made to data where the same protocol has been used.

Bench Press Muscular Endurance Test (aka. The NFL-225 Test)

Because of the strong association between maximal muscular strength and muscular endurance, repetitions to failure performed with an absolute load are commonly used to predict 1RM performance, especially in the bench press (Mayhew et al., 1999; Mayhew et al., 2002). Because performing bench press repetitions to failure with 225 lbs (102.3 kg) has been used extensively within the National Football League (NFL), it is commonly referred to as the NFL-225 test (Mayhew et al., 2002). Interestingly, Mayhew et al. (1999) reported a coefficient of determination (r^2) of 92%, although they noted a higher standard error of the estimate (SEE) when predicting 1RM performance, based on repetitions to failure when athletes could complete ≥10 repetitions (SEE = 17.1 lb) compared to when <10 repetitions (SEE = 11.1 lb) could be performed, with similar trends presented by Brechue and Mayhew (2009) and Mann et al. (2012). The prediction equations of Mayhew et al. (1999, 2002) are provided here:

$$1RM(lbs) = 226.7 + 7.1(repetitions\ at\ 225\ lbs)$$

Or

$$1RM(kg) = 102.3 + 3.23(repetitions\ at\ 102.3\ kg)$$

Hetzler et al. (2010) adapted the equations to take anthropometric data into account; however, this still resulted in similar predictive ability (r^2 = 0.87–0.90; 87–90%) for 1RM performance. Mann et al. (2014) also reported high reliability (ICC >0.98) and low variability (CV% <9.0) for the NFL-225 test. However, they also reported a high smallest worthwhile difference of >21.8–25.7%, which likely increases in stronger athletes who can perform a higher number of repetitions (Mayhew et al., 1999; Mayhew et al., 2002; Brechue and Mayhew, 2009; Mann et al., 2014). However, if not predicting 1RM performance, the smallest worthwhile change was three repetitions which may lead to inappropriate load selection (Mann et al., 2014).

Testing Protocol

With an absolute load of 225 lbs/102.3 kg, a minimum level of strength in the bench press is essential prior to attempting the NFL-225 test. To perform the test, athletes should warm up by performing the bench press, using progressively increasing loads, while the repetitions decrease, to ensure that the neuromuscular system is appropriately prepared for the test, but not in a state of fatigue. To perform the bench press, the athlete should lie on a bench, with their feet on the floor and their buttocks and

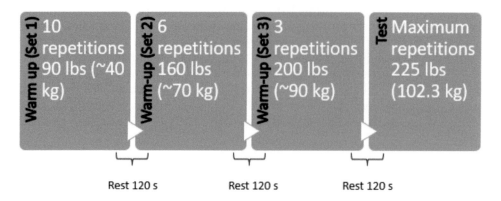

Rest 120 s   Rest 120 s   Rest 120 s

Figure 8.5 Standardized sequence for the NFL-225 test.

shoulders in contact with the bench. The bar should be grasped with a grip slightly wider (15–35 cm) than shoulder width (Mayhew et al., 2002), the bar should start above the shoulders and be lowered in a controlled manner until it touches the sternum, followed by a controlled press back to full extension of the elbows, with the bar moving in a slight arc. Once the warm-up is completed, the athletes should perform as many repetitions as possible without pausing at the top of the movement. Once the athlete can no longer complete a full repetition, the test is complete (Figure 8.5). If, during the final repetition, the full range of motion cannot be completed, this repetition should not be included.

Summary

Try performing some (i.e., those that you have the ability to perform competently and safely) of the muscular endurance tests and compare your performance to some of the published "norms," either within this chapter or from some of the published research and see how you fair against different populations.

Also consider performing a 1RM bench press and the NFL-225 test (for those who can) across your class and then evaluate the association between maximal strength and muscular endurance. In most cases, increases in strength are associated with an increase in endurance and vice versa.

References

Barringer, N. D., Mckinnon, C. J., O'brien, N. C. & Kardouni, J. R. 2019. Relationship of strength and conditioning metrics to success on the army ranger physical assessment test. *J Strength Cond Res*, 33(4), 958–64.

Baumgartner, T. A., Oh, S., Chung, H. & Hales, D. 2002. Objectivity, reliability, and validity for a revised push-up test protocol. *Meas Phys Edu Exerc Sci*, 6, 225–42.

Beckham, G. K., Olmeda, J. J., Flores, A. J., Echeverry, J. A., Campos, A. F. & Kim, S. B. 2018. Relationship between maximum pull-up repetitions and first repetition mean concentric velocity. *J Strength Cond Res*, 32(7), 1831–37.

Bianco, A., Jemni, M., Thomas, E., Patti, A., Paoli, A., Roque, J. R., Palma, A., Mammina, C. & Tabacchi, G. 2015. A systematic review to determine reliability and usefulness of the field-based test batteries for the assessment of physical fitness in adolescents – The ASSO project. *Int J Occup Med Environ Health*, 28, 445–78.

Brechue, W. F. & Mayhew, J. L. 2009. Upper-body work capacity and 1RM prediction are unaltered by increasing muscular strength in college football players. *J Strength Cond Res*, 23(9), 2477–86.

Cantell, M., Crawford, S. G. & Doyle-Baker, P. K. 2008. Physical fitness and health indices in children, adolescents and adults with high or low motor competence. *Hum Mov Sci*, 27, 344–62.

Castro-Piñero, J., Artero, E. G., España-Romero, V., Ortega, F. B., Sjöström, M., Suni, J. & Ruiz, J. R. 2010. Criterion-related validity of field-based fitness tests in youth: A systematic review. *Br J Sports Med*, 44, 934.

Fernandes, J. F. T., Lamb, K. L., Clark, C. C. T., Moran, J., Drury, B., Garcia-Ramos, A. & Twist, C. 2021. Comparison of the FitroDyne and GymAware rotary encoders for quantifying peak and mean velocity during traditional multijointed exercises. *J Strength Cond Res*, 35, 1760–5.

Hashim, A., Ariffin, A., Hashim, A. T. & Yusof, A. B. 2018. Reliability and validity of the 90° push-ups test protocol. *Int J Sci Res Manag*, 6, PE-2018-01-05.

Haugen, T., Høigaard, R. & Seiler, S. 2013. Normative data of BMI and physical fitness in a Norwegian sample of early adolescents. *Scand J Public Health2*, 42, 67–73.

Hetzler, R. K., Schroeder, B. L., Wages, J. J., Stickley, C. D. & Kimura, I. F. 2010. Anthropometry increases 1 repetition maximum predictive ability of NFL-225 test for division IA college football players. *J Strength Cond Res*, 24(6), 1429–39.

Lockie, R. G., Dawes, J. J., Orr, R. M. & Dulla, J. M. 2020. Recruit fitness standards from a large law enforcement agency: Between-class comparisons, percentile rankings, and implications for physical training. *J Strength Cond Res*, 34(4), 934–41.

Lubans, D. R., Morgan, P., Callister, R., Plotnikoff, R. C., Eather, N., Riley, N. & Smith, C. J. 2011. Test–retest reliability of a battery of field-based health-related fitness measures for adolescents. *J Sports Sci*, 29, 685–93.

Mann, J. B., Stoner, J. D. & Mayhew, J. L. 2012. NFL-225 test to predict 1RM bench press in NCAA division I football players. *J Strength Cond Res*, 26(10), 2623–31.

Mann, J. B., Ivey, P. J., Brechue, W. F. & Mayhew, J. L. 2014. Reliability and smallest worthwhile difference of the NFL-225 test in NCAA division I football players. *J Strength Cond Res*, 28(5), 1427–32.

Mayhew, J. L., Ware, J. S., Bemben, M. G., Wilt, B., Ward, T. E., Farris, B., Juraszek, J. O. E. & Slovak, J. P. 1999. The NFL-225 test as a measure of bench press strength in college football players. *J Strength Cond Res*, 13(2), 130–34.

Mayhew, J. L., Ware, J. S., Cannon, K., Corbett, S., Chapman, P. P., Bemben, M. G., Ward, T. E., Farris, B., Juraszek, J. & Slovak, J. P. 2002. Validation of the NFL-225 test for predicting 1-RM bench press performance in college football players. *J Sports Med Phys Fitness*, 42(3), 304–8.

McManis, B. G., Baumgartner, T. A. & Wuest, D. A. 2000. Objectivity and reliability of the 90° push-up test. *Meas Phys Educ Exerc Sci*, 4, 57–67.

Ojeda, Á. H., Maliqueo, S. G. & Barahona-Fuentes, G. 2020. Validity and reliability of the muscular fitness test to evaluate body strength-resistance. *Apunts Sports Med*, 55, 128–36.

Pate, R. R., Burgess, M. L., Woods, J. A., Ross, J. G. & Baumgartner, T. 1993. Validity of field tests of upper body muscular strength. *Res Q Exerc Sport*, 64, 17–24.

Plowman, S. A. 2013. Muscular strength, endurance, and flexibility assessments. In: Plowman, S. A. & Meredith, M. D. (eds). *Fitnessgram/Activitygram Reference Guide*. 4th ed. Dallas, Texas: The Cooper Institute.

Quinney, H. A., Smith, D. J. & Wenger, H. A. 1984. A field test for the assessment of abdominal muscular endurance in professional ice hockey players. *J Orthop Sports Phys Ther*, 6, 30–3.

Sanchez-Moreno, M., Parejo-Blanco, F., Diaz-Cueli, D. & Gonzalez-Badillo, J. J. 2016. Determinant factors of pull-up performance in trained athletes. *J Sports Medicine Phys Fitness*, 56, 825–33.

Sparling, P. B., Millard-Stafford, M. & Snow, T. K. 1997. Development of a cadence curl-up test for college students. *Res Q Exerc Sport*, 68, 309–16.

Vanderburgh, P. M. & Edmonds, T. 1997. The effect of experimental alterations in excess mass on pull-up performance in fit young men. *J Strength Cond Res*, 11(4), 203–33.

Weakley, J., Morrison, M., García-Ramos, A., Johnston, R., James, L. & Cole, M. H. 2021. The validity and reliability of commercially available resistance training monitoring devices: A systematic review. *Sports Med*, 51, 443–502.

Wood, H. M. & Baumgartner, T. A. 2004. Objectivity, reliability, and validity of the bent-knee push-up for college-age women. *Meas Phys Educ Exerc Sci*, 8, 203–12.

Woods, J. A., Pate, R. R. & Burgess, M. L. 1992. Correlates to performance on field tests of muscular strength. *Pediatr Exerc Sci*, 4, 302–11.

9 Anaerobic Capacity

Joshua Miller

Part 1: Introduction

The ability to regenerate adenosine triphosphate (ATP) is necessary, no matter how long a sporting event lasts. Certain activities may take a few seconds to accomplish the goal or hours depending upon the type of activity that is being performed. However, individuals will benefit from the regeneration of ATP through non-oxidative pathways in training or competition (Hermansen, 1969). Upon the beginning of movement, ATP is immediately catabolized to release energy for movement to occur. Once ATP is broken down, regeneration of ATP must occur to continue the event. The ability to regenerate ATP via non-oxidative pathways is called anaerobic metabolism. Anaerobic metabolism occurs in the cytoplasm of the cell and regenerates ATP without oxygen (O_2) being present. The human body has two anaerobic energy systems – the phosphagen (ATP-PC) system and glycolysis. Medbø et al. (1988) suggest that the energy derived from intramuscular phosphagen stores and anaerobic glycolysis is limited. This limitation may suggest that the anaerobic systems have a maximal capacity. Anaerobic capacity may be beneficial for athletes that participate in specific events like 400- to 1500-m running, 200- to 400-m swimming, 1- to 4-kilometre (km) cycling, and 2000-m rowing.

Energy Systems

It does not matter whether the sporting event or training protocol is one of power or endurance, the energy demands are met through the degradation of ATP. Unfortunately, there is a limited storage capacity of ATP within the muscle itself (< few seconds). To continue the work necessary to accomplish the play or repetitions, ATP must be regenerated via aerobic or anaerobic pathways.

The ATP-PCr system is the simplest of the energy systems. The body stores a small amount of ATP directly; the cells contain another high-energy phosphate molecule that stores energy called phosphocreatine (may also be called creatine phosphate, PCr). This pathway involves the donation of the inorganic phosphate (P_i) from PCr to adenosine diphosphate (ADP) to reform ATP via the enzyme creatine kinase (CK). The amount of PCr stored allows for approximately 3 seconds to 15 seconds of exercise (Brooks et al., 2004). The second anaerobic energy system in the regeneration of ATP utilizes the breakdown of glucose or glycogen stored in the muscle. This pathway is a little more complex than the ATP-PCr system and it is called glycolysis. Metabolism of glucose anaerobically results in 10–11 enzymatic steps that will

DOI: 10.4324/9781003186762-9

result in the regeneration of 2 or 3 ATP based upon the starting molecule of glucose or glycogen, respectively, and the production of lactic acid. The glycolytic pathway is the predominant energy system for supramaximal exercise lasting from 6 second to 1 minute, and then the major contributor is the aerobic energy system for the regeneration of ATP (Medbø and Tabata, 1989; Withers et al., 1991). All energy systems work together during exercise so that no one energy system works alone. The contributions of the energy systems are based upon the intensity and duration of the training protocol or sporting event.

Fatigue and Lactate

During supramaximal efforts, a lack of O_2 availability causes there to be an increase in lactate production via glycolysis. Blood lactate (BLa-) concentration represents the lactate produced in the muscle, transportation of the lactate from the muscles to the blood, and removal of the lactate from the blood (Gollnick and Hermansen, 1973). During supramaximal exercise, BLa- can be measured at the end of exercise to see intensity of the exercise completed (Chwalbinska-Moneta et al., 1989). It was once believed that the accumulation of BLa- caused muscle fatigue; however, that belief has been debunked (Bangsbo and Juel, 2006; Lamb and Stephenson, 2006). It is now believed that supramaximal exercise may inhibit both contractile and energy-producing processes (Osborne and Minahan, 2013).

Measurement of Anaerobic Capacity

Indirect measurements have been developed to reflect the ATP production during anaerobic activities. These techniques can be in the measurement of the oxygen deficit, BLa- concentrations after exercise, and the total amount of work completed during a short-bout of exercise. The best test for measurement of total work completed during short bouts of exercise is the Wingate Anaerobic test (WAnT) (Inbar et al., 1976; Weber et al., 2006; Green & Dawson, 1993). The total work completed, and the mean power output achieved during the WAnT has been used to predict anaerobic capacity (Zupan et al., 2009). Accumulated O_2 deficit has been used for the past several decades to quantify anaerobic ATP production during supramaximal exercise to exhaustion (Karlsson and Saltin, 1970). This test incorporates a laboratory-based test that measures the VO_2-power output relationship. The VO_2-power output relationship appears to be linear within a range of different exercise intensity (Medbø et al., 1988). Once the VO_2-power output relationship has been determined, the O_2 demand for supramaximal exercise can be extrapolated via linear regression modelling. The accumulated O_2 deficit represents the total energy required to fuel the supramaximal exercise bout and is the product of O_2 demand and exercise duration. The accumulated O_2 deficit can be calculated as the difference between the accumulated O_2 demand and the total VO_2. The accumulated O_2 deficit is measured in O_2 equivalents and represents the energy that is created from anaerobic intramuscular phosphagens (ATP and PCr) as well as ATP from glycolysis. The maximal accumulated O_2 deficit (MAOD) is the maximal value the accumulated O_2 deficit reaches during supramaximal exercise (Medbø et al., 1988) and can be determined via the MAOD test (Medbø et al., 1988).

The laboratory section will take the coach through determining anaerobic capacity via the MAOD, WAnT, and the Margaria-Kalamen step test.

Part 2: Maximal Accumulated Oxygen Deficit (MAOD)

The MAOD test is considered the gold standard test to determine anaerobic capacity (Noordhof et al., 2010); Tabata et al., 1997). However, Bangsbo (1992, 1996, 1998) is strongly opposed to its validity. With the controversy, the MAOD still remains the best measure for anaerobic capacity. The MAOD test can be performed via a treadmill or cycle ergometer. No matter the mode of the test, two main assumptions are made:

- The mechanical efficiency of supramaximal work is identical to that for submaximal work.
- The O_2 or energy demand for supramaximal exercise can be determined by extrapolation of the VO_2-power output relationship determined from VO_2 measured during several submaximal exercise bouts (Osborne and Minahan, 2013).

In the literature, the number, duration, and intensity of the submaximal exercise bouts have varied for measurement of MAOD (Medbø et al., 1988; Medbø and Tabata, 1989, 1993). These bouts were at least 10 bouts with a duration of 10 minutes for the determination of the VO_2-power output relationship. In the original study, Medbø et al. (1988) and recently Faina et al. (1997) and Calbet et al. (1997) used one supramaximal bout of exercise to determine the MAOD. Therefore, there is no universal protocol for the MAOD.

MAOD – Cycling

Testing Protocol

Determination of the VO_2-power output relationship is required to calculate the MAOD on the athlete. To do so, an athlete should complete a VO_{2max} test in which VO_2 can be measured during different power outputs. The protocol should consist of four to five submaximal VO_2 values during a continuous step cycling protocol or during the first stages of an incremental test to determine VO_{2max} (see Chapter 10).

The testing protocol begins with a warm-up period. This should be a power output that is not too taxing on the rider. Upon completion of the warm-up, the power output will be increased to 80–90% of VO_{2max}. Each stage will last 5 minutes, and power output will be increased at a set value of 30–50 W depending upon the abilities of the athlete. Throughout the testing, the athlete will be wearing a mouthpiece or mask for VO_2 analysis via the metabolic cart.

Upon completion of the test, the averaging of the final 2 minutes of each stage will be calculated and plotted on a graph for inclusion of the VO_2-power output relationship (Figure 9.1). This portion of the test will be completed prior to MAOD testing to determine peak VO_2 and establish the power output achieved at VO_{2max}.

A separate test should be completed to determine MAOD. This test will require the athlete to complete the test that corresponds to a power output of 120% of the power output achieved during the maximal test. A similar warm-up can be completed prior to the start of the test. The athlete will be wearing the mouthpiece or mask as they were during the maximal test. The test will begin with 0 W at a pedal cadence of 85 to 90 revolutions·min^{-1} (rpm). The power output associated to 120% of peak power output will be applied and VO_2 will be measured throughout the test. Verbal encouragement will be needed during the test. The test will be terminated when a pedal cadence of 40 rpm can no longer be maintained. Immediately, upon completion of the test, record the exact time of the test and allow for a cool-down to occur.

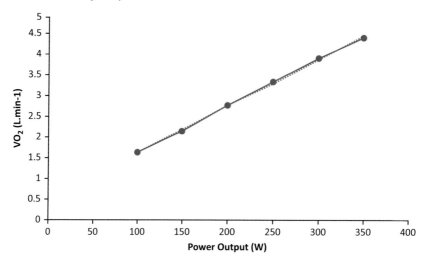

Figure 9.1 Plot of VO₂-power output relationship with linear equation.

Data Analysis

Prior to determining MAOD, a couple of data points are needed to be determined. Peak power output needs to be known from the maximal test, and determination of the VO_2-power output relationship needs to be determined (Table 9.1).

Step 1: The VO_2 for each submaximal stage will be plotted against power output to determine the linear relationship.

$y = a + bx$, where

y = oxygen demand in liters,
x = power output in watts,
b = slope of the regression line (0.0115), and
a = y-intercept of regression line (0.5135).
So, $y = 0.5135 + 0.115x$

Thus, the oxygen demand for a power output equal to 120% of the power output achieved at peak VO_2 (450 W × 1.20 = 540 W) is 6.55 L·min⁻¹.

Table 9.1 Values of the VO_2-power output relationship (cycling).

Power Output (W)	Time (min)	Stage	VO_2 ($L \cdot min^{-1}$)
100	0–5	1	1.67
150	5–10	2	2.2
200	10–15	3	2.83
250	15–20	4	3.41
300	20–25	5	4.0
30 min rest period			
350	0–5	6	4.5

Maximal power output is 450 W.

Table 9.2 O_2 uptake values obtained during 120% of peak power output test.

Power Output (W)	Time (min:s)	VO_2 $(L \cdot min^{-1})$	VO_2 $(L \cdot s^{-1})$
540	0–0:30	2.14	1.07
540	0:30–1:00	4.5	2.25
540	1:00–1:30	4.92	2.46
540	1:30–2:00	5.18	2.59
540	2:00–2:30	5.4	2.7

Step 2: Need to determine the MAOD: The total O_2 demand (accumulated O_2 demand) of the constant load test can be calculated by multiplying the O_2 demand by the duration of the test.

O_2 demand = 6.55 $L \cdot min^{-1}$

Duration of test = 2.5 minutes

So accumulated O_2 demand = 6.55 $L \cdot min^{-1} \times 2.5$ min = 16.375 L

The total O_2 consumption (accumulated O_2 uptake) measured via the metabolic cart during the test can be calculated by converting each VO_2 value from $L \cdot min^{-1}$ to $L \cdot 30$ s^{-1} (Table 9.2) and the sum of the values:

Accumulated O_2 uptake = 11.07 L.

The accumulated O_2 deficit is calculated by subtracting the accumulated O_2 uptake from the accumulated O_2 deficit:

$16.375 - 11.07 = 5.31$ $LO_2eq \cdot kg^{-1}$

Then, subtract 9% of the accumulated O_2 deficit to account for O_2 stores:

$5.31 \times 9\% = 4.83$ $LO_2eq \cdot kg^{-}$

Data Interpretation (Brief explanation of key variables, supported by an example case study, with additional examples that the reader can work through. Also include other tests and associated variables that may provide additional insight.)

Wingate Anaerobic Test (WAnT)

The Wingate Anaerobic Test (WAnT) was initially designed for adolescents (Cumming, 1972) and then became popular for adults in the late 1970s (Bar-Or, 1978). The WAnT has been used more than any other test for anaerobic capacity and supramaximal exercise (Ayalon et al., 1974). The WAnT was initially designed as a leg cycle ergometer test, but it has been adapted for arm-crank ergometry to test upper body anaerobic capacity. It fulfilled the need for a test to measure anaerobic power.

This anaerobic test can determine an athlete's peak power output (PP), mean anaerobic power (MAP), total work, and fatigue index (FI). Peak power is the highest power output achieved over the first 5 seconds of the test; in comparison, MAP refers to the average power during the entire 30 sec of the test. Total work is calculated as the product of the total number of pedal revolutions completed and the force or resistance during the test. The FI measures the rate of power decrease from the point of peak anaerobic power to the finish of the test. The FI can be used to estimate the percentage of fast-twitch muscle fibres in the vastus lateralis (Bar-Or et al., 1980).

Wingate Anaerobic Test (WAnT)

Methodological Information

The test has been demonstrated to be a reliable test for peak (PP) and mean (MP) power output. Reliability coefficients in a test-retest range from about 0.90 to 0.98 for peak and mean power output (Inbar et al., 1976; Evans and Quinney, 1981).

Testing Protocol

The Wingate test requires the athlete to pedal or arm-crank for 30 seconds at maximal speed against a constant resistance for males and females (Table 9.3) and sport-specific athletes (Table 9.4). This resistance is predetermined percentage of the individual's body mass that would allow for a noticeable development of fatigue to occur within the initial few seconds of the test.

Individuals will perform a warm-up on the cycle ergometer for approximately 5 minutes with approximately 0.5–1.0 kg of resistance. Prior to starting the warm-up, the athlete's seat height should be set with his knee bent approximately 10 degrees at the bottom of the pedal stroke. During minutes 2–4, the athlete will increase the pedal cadence above 100 $rev \cdot min^{-1}$ for 10 sec and then return to normal. Upon completion of the warm-up, the athlete will be reminded to increase his pedal cadence as fast as possible (>120 $rev \cdot min^{-1}$) prior to the beginning of the test. Once the pedal cadence is achieved, the resistance will be lowered, and the clock will begin counting down from 30 seconds. At the end of the test, the resistance will be removed, and the athlete should continue to pedal against 0.5–1.0 kg of resistance for a few minutes to aid in recovery. Verbal encouragement may be needed during the test for a maximal effort.

Table 9.3 The optimal load for the Wingate test in males and females.

Subjects	Limb	Force (kp/kg)	Work (J/rev/kg)	Reference
		Adult males		
Sedentary	Legs	0.075	4.41	Ayalon et al. (1974)
Active and athletes	Legs	0.098	5.76	Evans and Quinney (1981)
Phys. Ed. Students	Legs	0.087	5.13	Dotan and Bar-Or (1983)
Soldiers	Legs	0.094	5.53	Patton et al. (1985)
Phys. Ed. Students	Arms	0.062	3.62	Dotan and Bar-Or (1983)
		Adult females		
Phys. Ed. Students	Legs	0.085	5.04	Dotan and Bar-Or (1983)
Phys. Ed. Students	Arms	0.048	2.82	Dotan and Bar-Or (1983)

Kp = kilopond; kg = kilogram; J/rev/kg = joules per revolution per kilogram.

Table 9.4 The optimal load for the Wingate test in male and female athletes.

Sport	Force (kp/kg)	Reference
Football – NCAA DI	0.083	Seiler et al. (1990)
Kickboxing – Elite	Not listed	Zabukovec and Tiidus (1995)
Runners – Middle Distance	Load based upon Force-Velocity test	Granier et al. (1995)
Sprinters – Elite	4–7 kg	Crielaard and Pirnary (1981)
Sprinters – Elite	Load based upon Force-Velocity test	Granier et al. (1995)
Soccer – Youth	0.075	Vanderford et al. (2004)
Soccer – US National	0.075	Mangine et al., 1990
Speed Skating – Elite	$(0.092 + 0.112 \text{ kp} \cdot \text{kg}^{-1}$ (BM)	Smith and Roberts (1991)
Tennis – NCAA	0.075	Kraemer et al. (2003)
Hockey – NCAA DIII	0.086 (male), 0.075 (female)	Janot et al. (2015)

kp = kilopond; kg = kilogram.

Data Analysis

During the 30 seconds of testing, the three performance variables are measured: PP, MP, and FI.

Here is an example of data from a male who weighs 85 kg while performing the Wingate test on a Monark cycle ergometer (Figure 9.2, Tables 9.5–9.7).

Peak power (PP) = Resistance (kg) × distance around flywheel (Monark = 6 m) × total # of revolutions in 5 seconds

$$= 6.4 \text{ kg of resistance} \times 6 \text{ m} \times 15 \text{ revolutions} = 576 \text{ kgm} \cdot 5 \text{ sec}^{-1}$$
$$= 576 \text{ kgm} \cdot 5 \text{ sec}^{-1} \times 12 = 6912 \text{ kgm} \cdot \text{min}^{-1}/6.12 = \underline{1129.4 \text{ W}}$$

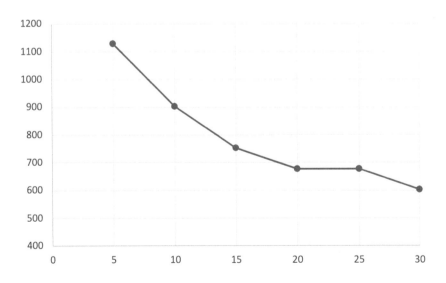

Figure 9.2 Graphic representation of the Wingate test.

Table 9.5 Time representation of the Wingate test.

Time (sec)	Resistance	Distance	Revolutions	Work (kg m · 5 sec⁻¹)
0–5	6.4	6	15	576
5–10	6.4	6	12	460.8
10–15	6.4	6	10	384
15–20	6.4	6	9	345.6
20–25	6.4	6	9	345.6
25–30	6.4	6	8	307.2
Total			63	2419.2 kg m · 30 sec⁻¹

Sec = seconds; kg m · 5 sec⁻¹ = kilogram meters per 5 seconds; kg m · 30 sec⁻¹ = kilogram meters per 30 seconds.

Mean power (MAP) = Resistance (kg) × distance around flywheel (Monark = 6 m) × total # of revolutions

$$= 6.4 \text{ kg of resistance} \times 6 \text{ m} \times 63 \text{ revolutions} = 2419.2 \text{ kgm} \cdot 30 \text{ sec}^{-1}$$

$$= 2419.2 \text{ kgm} \cdot 30 \text{ sec}^{-1} \times 2 = 4838.4 \text{ kgm} \cdot \text{min}^{-1}/6.12 = \underline{790.6 \text{ W}}$$

Fatigue Index (FI) = ((Peak power output − minimum power output)/Peak power output) × 100

$$= \left(\left(576 \text{ kgm} \cdot 5 \text{ sec}^{-1} - 307.2 \text{ kgm} \cdot 5 \text{ sec}^{-1} \right)/576 \text{ kgm} \cdot 5 \text{ sec}^{-1} \right) \times 100 = \underline{46.7}$$

% fast-twitch = (Fatigue index − 19)/0.5

$$= (46.7 - 19)/0.5$$

$$= \underline{55.4\% \textit{ fast-twitch muscle}}$$

Data Interpretation

Comparison of the athlete's PP and MP can be made upon completion of the test.

Table 9.6 Examples of PP and MP for specific sport populations as well as male and female.

Sport	Gender	Peak Power	Mean Power	Reference
Basketball – NCAA DI	F	663 + 98	498 + 51	LaMonte et al. (1999)
Bobsled – US National	M	1005 + 90	796 + 60	Osbeck et al. (1996)
Football – NCAA DI	M	1189 + 130	874 + 102	Seiler et al. (1990)
Football – NCAA DIII	M	1894 + 140	1296 + 66	Hoffman et al. (2004)
Kickboxing – Elite	M	1360	761	Zabukovec and Tiidus (1995)
Runners – Middle Distance	M	842 + 123	578 + 65	Granier et al. (1995)
Softball – Masters	F	Not listed	406 + 56	Terbizan et al. (1996)

Table 9.7 Category for peak and mean anaerobic power and fatigue index for men and women.

Category	%ile	Peak Anaerobic Power				Mean Anaerobic Power				Fatigue Index	
		Men (N = 52)		Women (N = 50)		Men		Women		Men	Women
		Absolute (W)	Relative (W·kg⁻¹)	Absolute (W)	Relative (W·kg⁻¹)	Absolute (W)	Relative (W·kg⁻¹)	Absolute (W)	Relative (W·kg⁻¹)	(%)	(%)
Well above average	95	867	11.1	602	9.3	677	8.6	483	7.5	21	20
Above average	90	822	10.9	560	9.0	662	8.2	470	7.3	23	25
	85	807	10.6	530	8.9	631	8.1	437	7.1	27	25
	75	768	10.4	518	8.6	504	8.0	414	6.9	30	28
Average	70	757	10.2	505	8.5	600	7.9	410	6.8	31	29
	50	689	9.2	449	7.6	565	7.4	381	6.4	38	35
	30	656	8.5	399	6.9	530	7.0	353	6.0	43	40
Below average	25	646	8.3	396	6.8	521	6.8	347	5.9	45	42
	15	594	7.4	362	6.4	485	6.4	320	5.6	47	44
	10	570	7.1	353	6.0	471	6.0	306	5.3	52	47
Well below average	5	530	6.6	329	5.7	453	5.6	287	5.1	55	48
Mean		**700**	**9.2**	**455**	**7.6**	**563**	**7.3**	**381**	**6.4**	**38**	**35**
S.D.		95	1.4	81	1.2	67	0.9	56	0.7	10	8
Minimum		500	5.3	239	4.6	441	4.6	235	5.5	15	18
Maximum		927	11.9	623	10.6	711	9.1	529	8.1	58	49

Adapted from Maud and Schultz (1989).

Margaria-Kalamen Step Test

One of the most common anaerobic step tests performed by athletes and in clinical settings is the Margaria stair climb test (Margaria et al., 1966) and then modified by Kalamen (Kalamen 1968). The current version of the test is designed to test anaerobic power due to the extremely short duration (less than 5 sec) of the test. The energy system that contributes to the test is the phosphagen (ATP-PC) system (Margaria et al., 1966).

The Margaria-Kalamen step test is considered very reliable and has a test-retest reliability of r = 0.85 and a CV of < 4% (MacDougall et al., 1991). Safety is a key factor for this test and should be taken into consideration for an individual who is less experienced or shorter in height due to the difficulty of stepping three steps at a time.

Methodological Information

To perform this test, a running path of 6 m (19.7 ft) with at least 9 steps, each step is between 174 and 175 cm (68.5 and 68.9 in.) in height (Skinner et al., 2014). It may be beneficial to use an electronic switch mat, or photoelectric cell on steps three and nine to ensure accurate timing (Hoffman 2006), but if you do not have these types of equipment, a standard stopwatch can be used accurately (Skinner et al., 2014). The goal is to have the athlete run up the stairs as fast as possible by taking three steps at a time (Figure 9.3).

Testing Protocol

Prior to beginning the test, if electronic switches or photoelectric cells are unavailable, mark steps three and nine with tape or a cone. This will allow the coach with the stopwatch to start and stop the timer. Measure the height and distance of the steps

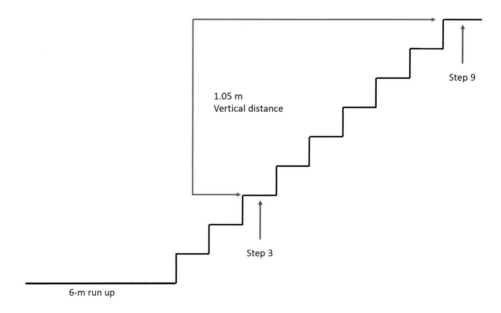

Figure 9.3 Margaria-Kalamen Step test illustration.

from step three to nine and convert to meters. Once the athlete is properly warmed up and understands the test procedures, have the athlete stand behind the start line 6 m before the steps. On "Go," the athlete should run as fast as possible to the stairs and take three steps at a time. The stopwatch will be started when the athlete steps on step three and stopped when he/she steps on the ninth step. Mark the time at the end of the test. Three trials will be completed and allow for at least 2–3 minutes for recovery between trials.

Data Analysis

Upon completion of the test, power can be calculated from the following equation:

$$\text{Power}\left(\text{kg} \cdot \text{m} \cdot \text{sec}^{-1}\right) = \left(\text{Body mass (kg)} \times \text{distance (m)}\right)/\text{time (sec)}$$

Where weight is the athlete's body mass in kilograms, distance is the vertical height between steps three and nine, and the time is the number of seconds it takes the athlete to run up steps three and nine.

Power can be converted to watts by multiplying the answer by 9.807, which is the equivalent to the normal acceleration due to gravity.

$$\text{Watts (W)} = \text{Power}\left(\text{kg} \cdot \text{m} \cdot \text{sec}^{-1}\right) \times 9.807$$

So, using the numbers from Figure 9.3 for vertical distance, an athlete who weighs 95 kg, and completes the test in 1.5 second power, is determined as follows:

Power (kg m sec^{-1}) = (weight (kg) × distance (m))/time (sec)

$$= ((95 \text{ kg} \times 1.05 \text{ m}) / 1.5 \text{ Sec}^{-1}$$

$$= 66.5 \text{ kg} \cdot \text{m} \cdot \text{sec}^{-1}, \text{ convert to W,}$$

$$= 66.5 \text{ kg} \cdot \text{m} \cdot \text{sec}^{-1} \times 9.807 = \underline{652.2 \text{ W}}$$

Data Interpretation

Comparison to normative data can determine the athlete's abilities (Table 9.8). This normative data table is in watts.

Table 9.8 Normative values for the Margaria-Kalamen stair step sprint test.

Category	15–20 y M	15–20 y F	20–30 y M	20–30 y F	30–40 y M	30–40 y F	40–50 y M	40–50 y F	50+ y M	50+ y F
Excellent	2197	1789	2059	1648	1648	1226	1226	961	961	736
Good	1840	1487	1722	1379	1379	1036	1036	810	809	604
Average	1839	1486	1721	1378	1378	1035	1035	809	809	603
Fair	1466	1182	1368	1094	1094	829	829	642	641	476
Poor	1108	902	1040	834	834	637	637	490	490	373

Kalamen (1968), Margaria et al. (1966).

Name: _____

Body Mass (kg): _____

Seconds	Resistance	×	6	×	Revolutions	=	Work (kgm·5-sec^{-1})
0–5	_____	×	6	×	_____	=	_____
5–10	_____	×	6	×	_____	=	_____
10–15	_____	×	6	×	_____	=	_____
15–20	_____	×	6	×	_____	=	_____
20–25	_____	×	6	×	_____	=	_____
25–30	_____	×	6	×	_____	=	_____
0–30		×	6	×		=	kgm·30-sec^{-1}

Resistance (_____ × kg of body mass) = _____ kg
Use Table 9.× to determine % of body mass for the athlete.

Peak Power (PP) = Resistance (kg) × distance around flywheel (Monark = 6m) × total # of revolutions in 5-sec
PP = _____ kgm·5-sec^{-1} × 12 / 6.12 = _____ watts

Mean power (MAP) = Resistance (kg) × distance around flywheel (Monark = 6m) × total # of revolutions
MAP = _____ kgm·30-sec^{-1} × 12 / 6.12 = _____ watts

Minimum Power (MP) = Resistance (kg) × distance around flywheel (Monark = 6m) × lowest total # of revolutions in 5-sec
MP = _____ kgm·5-sec^{-1} × 12 / 6.12 = _____ watts

Fatigue Index (FI) = ((PP output – MP output) / PP output) × 100
FI = ((_____ – _____) / _____) × 100 = _____%

Percent fast-twitch muscle (% FT) = (Fatigue index – 19) / 0.5
% FT = (_____ – 19) / 0.5 = _____

Insert Table to graphically display Wingate test.

Evaluation / Comments:
_____
_____
_____
_____

Figure 9.4 Wingate test data sheet.

Laboratory Task: Are You Ready for Exercise?

Complete all three tests to determine anaerobic capacity and discuss methods to increase an athlete's anaerobic capacity for certain sports (Figures 9.4 and 9.5)

Summary

This chapter dealt with the assessment of anaerobic capacity and power in individuals. The energy systems that are impacted primarily have been described and the

Name: _____   Gender: _____

Body Mass (kg): _____   Height (cm): _____

Vertical Distance, between steps 3 and 9 (meters): _____

Time (sec): _____ (Trial 1)

Time (sec): _____ (Trial 2)

Time (sec): _____ (Trial 3)

Calculate the power associated with the Margaria Kalamen test:

Power (kg·m·sec^{-1}) = (Body mass (kg) × distance (m)) / time (sec)

Power (kg·m·sec^{-1}) = (_____ (kg) × _____ (m)) / _____ (sec) = _____ kg·m·sec^{-1}

Convert power to watts:

Watts (w) = Power (kg·m·sec^{-1}) × 9.807

Watts (w) = _____ (kg·m·sec^{-1}) × 9.807 = _____ w

Evaluation / Comments:
_____
_____
_____
_____

Figure 9.5 Margaria-Kalamen step data sheet.

protocols should be followed to test the immediate and glycolytic energy systems. Testing strategy for the anaerobic systems should last less than 10, 30, and 90 seconds in order to maximally address the physiological characteristics maximally. The most frequently used anaerobic tests have been described and reference values for athletes have been included for comparison to the individual being tested.

References

Ayalon, A., Inbar, O. & Bar-Or, O. 1974. Relationships among measurements of explosive strength and anaerobic power. In: Nelson, R. C. & Moorehouse, C. A. (eds). *International Series on Sports Sciences*, Vol. I, Biomechanics IV, 527–32. Baltimore, MD: University Park Press.

Bangsbo, J. 1992. Is the O$_2$ deficit an accurate quantitative measure of the anaerobic energy prdcution during intense exercise? *J Appl Physiol*, 73, 1207–9.

Bansgbo, J. 1996. Oxygen deficit: A measure of the anaerobic energy production intense exercise? *Can J Appl Physiol*, 21, 350–63.

Bangsbo, J. 1998. Quantification of anaerobic energy production during intense exercise. *Med Sci Sports Exer*, 30, 47–52.

Bangsbo, J. & Juel, C. 2006. Counterpoint: Lactic acid accumulation is an advantage/disadvantage during muscle activity. *J Appl Physiol*, 100, 1412–3.

Bar-Or, O. 1978. A new anaerobic capacity test: Characteristics applications. *Proceedings of the 21st World Congress in Sports Medicine at Brasilia*.

Bar-Or, O., Dotan, R., Inbar, O., Rothstein, A., Karlsson, J. & Tesch, P. 1980. Anaerobic capacity and muscle fiber type distribution in man. *Int J Sports Med*, 1, 82–5.

Brooks, G. A., Fahey, T. D. & Baldwin, K. M. 2004. *Exercise Physiology: Human Bioenergetics and Its Applicatio*, 4th ed. New York, NY: McGraw-Hill.

Calbet, J. A., Chavarren, J. & Dorado, C. 1997. Fractional use of anaerobic capacity during a 30- and a 45-s Wingate test. *Eur J Appl Physiol Occup Physiol*, 76, 308–13.

Chwalbinska-Moneta, J., Roberg, R. A., Costill, D. C. & Fink, W. 1989. Threshold for muscle lactate accumulation during progressive exercise. *J Appl Physiol*, 66, 2710–6.

Crielaard, J. & Pirnay, F. 1981. Anaerobic and aerobic power of top athletes. *Euro J Appl Phys*, 47, 295–300.

Cumming, G. 1972. Correlation of athletic performance and aerobic power in 12- to 17-year-old children with bone age, calf muscle, total body potassium, heart volume and two indices of anaerobic power. *Proceedings of the Fourth International Symposium on Paediatric Work Physiology*, 109–34.

Dotan, R. & Bar-Or, O. 1983. Load optimization for the Wingate anaerobic test. *Euro J Appl Physiol*, 51, 409–17.

Evans, J. A. & Quinney, H. A. 1981. Determination of resistance settings for anaerobic power testing. *Can J Appl Sport Sci*, 6, 53–6.

Faina, M., Billat, V., Squadrone, R., De Anfelis, M., Koralsztein, J. P. & Dal Monte, A. 1997. Anaerobic contribution to the time to exhaustion at the minimal exercise intensity at which oxygen uptake occurs in elite cyclists, kayakists and swimmers. *Eur J Appl Physiol Occup Physiol*, 76, 13–20.

Gollnick, P. D. & Hermansen, L. 1973. Biochemical adaptation to exercise: Anaerobic metabolism. *Exer Sci Sports Rev*, 1, 1–43.

Granier, P., Mercier, B., Mercier, J. & Anselme, F. 1995. Aerobic and anaerobic contribution to Wingate test performance in sprint and middle-distance runners. *Euro J Appl Physiol*, 70, 58–65.

Green, S. & Dawson, B. 1993. Measurement of anaerobic capacities in humans. Definitions, limitations and unsolved problems. *Sports Med*, 15, 312–27.

Hermansen, L. 1969. Anaerobic energy release. *Med Sci Sports*, 1, 32–8.

Hoffman, J. R., 2006. *Norms for Fitness, Performance, and Health*. Champaign, IL: Human Kinetics.

Hoffman, J. R., Cooper, J., Wendell, M., Im, J. & Kang, J. 2004. Effects of β-hydroxy β-methylbutyrate on power performance and indices of muscle damage and stress during high intensity training. *J Strength Cond Res*, 18, 747–52.

Inbar, O., Dotan, R. & Bar-Or, O. 1976. Aerobic and anaerobic component of a thirty-second supramaximal cycling test. *Med Scie Sports*, 8, 51.

Janot, J. M., Beltz, N. M. & Dalleck, L. D. 2015. Multiple off-ice performance variables predict on-ice skating performance in male and female division III ice hockey players. *J Sports Sci Med*, 14, 522–9.

Kalamen, J. 1968. *Measurement of Maximum Muscle Power in Man*. Ohio: Ohio State University.

Karlsson, L. & Saltin, B. 1970. Lactate, ATP, and CP in working muscles during exhaustive exercise in man. *J Appl Physiol*, 29, 598–602.

Kraemer, W. J., Hakkinen, K., Triplett-McBride, T., Fry, A. C., Kozris, L. P., Ratamess, N. A., Bauer, J. E., Volek, J. S., McConnell, T., Newton, R. U., Gordon, S. E., Cummings, D., Hauth, J., Pullo, F., Lynch, J. M., Mazzetti, S. A. & Knuttgen, H. G. 2003. Physiological changes with periodized resistance training in women tennis players. *Med Sci Sport Exer*, 35, 157–68.

Lamb, G. D. & Stephenson, D. G. 2006. Point/Counterpoint: Lactic acid is an advantage/disadvantage during muscle activity. *J Appl Physiol*, 100, 1410–2.

LaMonte, M. J., McKinney, M. C., Quinn, S. M., Bainbridge, C. N. & Eisenman, P. A. 1999. Comparison of physical and physiological variables for female college basketball players. *J Strength Cond Res*, 13, 264–70.

MacDougall, J. D., Wenger, H. A. & Green, H. J. (eds). 1991. The purpose of physiological testing. In: *Physiological Testing of the High-Performance Athlete*, 1–6. Champaign, IL: Human Kinetics.

Mangine, R. E., Noyes, F. R., Mullen, M. P. & Baker, S. D. 1990. A physiological profile of the elite soccer athlete. *J Ortho Sports Phys Ther*, 12, 147–52.

Margaria, R., Aghemo, P. & Rovelli, E. 1966. Measurement of muscular power (anaerobic) in man. *J Appl Physiol*, 21, 1662–4.

Maud, P. J. & Schultz, B. B. 1989. Norms for the Wingate anaerobic test with comparison to another similar test. *Res Q Ex Sport*, 60, 144–51.

Medbø, J. I. & Tabata, I. 1989. Relative importance of aerobic and anaerobic energy release during short-lasting exhausting bicycle exercise. *J Appl Physiol*, 67, 1881–6.

Medbø, J. I. & Tabata, I. 1993. Anaerobic energy release in working muscle during 30 s to 3 min of exhausting bicycling. *J Appl Physiol*, 75, 1654–60.

Medbø, J. I., Mohn, A. C., Tabata, I., Bahr, R., Vaage, O. & Sejersted, O. M. 1988. Anaerobic capacity determined by maximal accumulated O_2 deficit. *J Appl*, 64, 50–60.

Noordhof, D. A., de Koning, J. J. & Foster, C. 2010. The maximal accumulated oxygen deficit method a valid and reliable measure of anaerobic capacity. *Sports Med*, 40, 285–302.

Osbeck, J., Maiorca, S. & Rundell, S. N. 1996. Validity of field testing to bobsled start performance. *J Strength Cond Res*, 10, 239–45.

Osborne, M. A. & Minahan, C. L. 2013. Anaerobic capacity. In: Tanner, R.K. & Gore, C.J. (eds). *Physiological Tests for Elite Athletes*, 2nd ed. 59–74. Champaign, IL: Human Kinetics.

Patton, J. F., Murphy, M. M. & Frederick, F. A. 1985. Maximal power outputs during the Wingate anaerobic test. *Int J Sports Med*, 6, 82–5.

Seiler, S., Taylor, M., Diana, R., Layes, J., Newton, P. & Brown, B. 1990. Assessing anaerobic power in collegiate football players. *J Appl Sport Sci Res*, 4, 9–15.

Skinner, T., Newton, R. U. & Haff, G. G. 2014. Neuromuscular strength, power, and strength endurance. In: Coombes, J.S., & Skinner, T. (eds). *ESSA's Student Manual for Health, Exercise, and Sport Assessment*. 133–73, Chatswood: Elsevier.

Smith, D. J. & Roberts, D. 1991. Aerobic, anaerobic and isokinetic measures of elite Canadian male and female speed skaters. *J Appl Sport Sci Res*, 5, 110–5.

Tabata, I., Irisawa, K., Kouzakia, M., Nishimura, K., Ogita, F. & Miyachi, M. 1997. Metabolic profile of high intensity intermittent exercises. *Med Sci Sports Exerc*, 29, 390–5.

Terbizan, D. J., Walders, M., Seljevold, P. & Schweigert, D. J. 1996. Physiological characteristics of masters women Fastpitch softball players. *J Strength Cond Res*, 10, 157–60.

Vanderford, M. L., Meyers, M. C., Skelly, W. A., Stewart, C. C. & Hamilton, K. L. 2004. Physiological and sport-specific skill response of Olympic youth soccer athletes. *J Strength Cond Res*, 18, 334–42.

Weber, C., Chia, M. & Inbar, O. 2006. Gender differences in anaerobic power of the arms and legs – A scaling issue. *Med Sci Sports Exer*, 38, 129–37.

Withers, R., Sherman, W., Clark, D., Essekbach, P. C., Bolan, S. R., Mackay, M. H. & Brinkman, M. 1991. Muscle metabolism during 30, 60, and 90s of maximal cycling on an air-braked ergometer. *Euro J Appl Physiol*, 63, 354–62.

Zabukovec, R. & Tiidus, P. M. 1995. Physiological and anthropometric profile of elite kickboxers. *J Strength Cond Res*, 9, 240–2.

Zupan, M. F., Arata, A. W., Dawson, L. H., Wile, A. L., Payn, T. L. & Hannon, M. E. 2009. Wingate anaerobic test peak power and anaerobic capacity classifications for men and women intercollegiate athletes. *J Strength Cond Res*, 23, 2598–604.

10 Aerobic Capacity Testing

Joshua Miller

Part 1: Introduction

Why Is Aerobic Capacity Necessary?

Depending upon the sport that is being played, cardiorespiratory fitness or aerobic capacity may not be the most ideal component that is assessed, but aerobic capacity is one of the most important components of fitness. Aerobic fitness is the ability to perform dynamic exercise that involves large muscle groups performing moderate-to-high intensity exercise for a prolonged time frame (ACSM, 2021). The energy that drives these large muscle groups need to create enough energy or adenosine triphosphate (ATP) to drive the excitation-contraction coupling processes from the hydrolysis of ATP. Due to the low concentration of stored ATP in the muscle, it must be regenerated by metabolic reactions at similar rates of consumption. The generation of ATP occurs via anaerobic and aerobic methods, with recovery between high-intensity activity (e.g. anaerobic metabolism) dependent on aerobic capacity. The focus of this chapter will be on the regeneration of ATP via aerobic mechanisms.

The rate at which aerobic metabolism can supply power is dependent upon the ability of the tissues to use oxygen (O_2) in breaking down fats and carbohydrates and the cardiopulmonary system to transport the O_2 to the muscles for use. In the laboratory, it may be difficult to isolate which system is the limiting factor, but measurement of aerobic capacity allows for the systems to be measured as one unit rather than separate ones.

Aerobic capacity should be considered an important part of testing athletes. Measurement of an individual's maximum oxygen uptake (VO_{2max}) is considered the gold standard measure of functional capacity of the cardiorespiratory system. VO_{2max} is the maximal rate of oxygen uptake (VO_2) during maximal exercise. This reflects the cardiovascular system's ability to pump blood to the body, the pulmonary system's ability to transfer oxygen (O_2) from the environment to the blood, and the blood's ability to transfer O_2 from the blood to the skeletal muscle for energy production to occur during exercise. The Fick equation describes the basic relationship between metabolism and cardiovascular function. Simply, the equation states that the O_2 consumed by the tissues is dependent upon the blood flow to the tissues and the amount extracted from the blood by the tissues. This equation can be applied to the whole body or to regional circulations. Oxygen consumption is the product of blood flow and the difference in concentration of O_2 in the blood between the arterial and venous systems known as the $(a-v)O_2$ difference. Whole body oxygen

DOI: 10.4324/9781003186762-10

consumption (VO_2) is calculated as the product of the cardiac output (Q) and the (a-v) O_2 difference. The Fick equation:

$$VO_2 = Q \times (a\text{-}v)O_2 \text{ difference}$$

Or the Fick equation can be written as:

$$VO_2 = [HR \times SV] \times (a\text{-}v)O_2 \text{ difference.}$$

Whereas HR is heart rate (the number of heart beats), and SV is stroke volume (volume of blood pumped per beat). This concept is one of the most important concepts in exercise physiology.

Energy Production

During all sports, no matter the length of time to complete the event, the breakdown (hydrolysis) of ATP or the prephosphorylation of adenosine diphosphate (ADP) is necessary to continue performance in the event. Traditionally, in sports lasting only seconds (i.e. weightlifting, sprinting, and throwing events), the phosphagen (ATP-PC) system enables the athlete to propel them to possible victory. During events that may last between 20 seconds and 2 minutes (i.e. events longer than 200 m, swimming medley events, and others), glycolysis will continue ATP production. During events that last longer than 2 minutes (i.e. marathon, cycling stage races, and others), oxidative phosphorylation will make more ATP via glucose and fatty acid metabolism. In all these events, all three energy systems are working together to allow the athlete to generate ATP production. An example of this can be demonstrated in a 400-m running event. Spencer and Gastin (2001) reported that aerobic metabolism accounted for approximately 43% of total energy production over the event.

The important difference between the ATP-PC system and oxidative phosphorylation is that the ATP-PC system rephosphorylates ADP via direct transfer of the phosphate group while oxidative phosphorylation relies on the oxidation of reducing equivalents in the electron-transport chain (ETC) of the mitochondria in the muscle. This requires O_2 to be present as an oxidizing agent when the energy transfer is being completed.

Why Assess Aerobic Capacity?

The assessment of aerobic capacity or VO_{2max} is the best objective laboratory measurement of cardiorespiratory fitness. In the seminal work of A. V. Hill in the 1920s (Hill et al., 1924; Hill and Lupton, 1923), the criterion measure of aerobic capacity is the VO_{2max}. As exercise intensity increases, oxygen (O_2) consumption will increase until the individual can no longer continue to perform (volitional fatigue and exercise must stop). As an individual performs endurance training, more O_2 can be delivered and used by the active muscles. Depending upon the training status of the individual undergoing training, an increase in VO_{2max} of 15% to 20% improvement has been demonstrated in untrained individual after completing 20 weeks of training. These improvements allow individuals to perform similar endurance activities for greater periods of time at a submaximal training intensity.

The current view may want to determine the parameters which reflect the fraction of maximal capacity that an athlete can use during prolonged exercise. This may enhance the protocol selected to determine functional capacity. This may include assessing critical power (CP) or critical velocity (CV), which is a direct measurement of the ability to perform mechanical work. CP or velocity represents the highest rate of energy turnover that can be maintained without drawing on the finite energy reserves (W') which would limit the ability to sustain high-energy work (Jones et al., 2010). This means that CP/CV could be a true indicator of aerobic functional capacity. In addition to the determination of VO_{2max}, there are several other physiological variables that can be measured during exercise that can be evaluated in athletes. This includes the lactate threshold (LT) (Wasserman and Mcilroy, 1964; Farrell et al., 1979; Tanaka et al., 1983), lactate turnpoint (LTP) (Davis and Gass, 1979; Davis et al., 1983), or respiratory compensation point (RCP) (Whipp et al., 1989), and maximal lactate steady state (MLSS) (Billat et al., 2003; Beneke et al., 2011).

Lactate Threshold

While performing aerobic capacity, the misnomer of measuring only the aerobic component is not correct. The test also incorporates measurement of the anaerobic system as well. As previously stated, all three energy systems work together to benefit the athlete performing their sport. As the test is being completed, the breakdown of free fatty acids will begin to decrease based upon the intensity of exercise being performed. As the intensity continues to increase, there will be a continual build-up of lactic acid. With the build-up of lactic acid within the muscle, the lactate and disassociated hydrogen ions will diffuse into the extracellular fluid to the plasma from the muscles.

Understanding the point at which lactate production is greater than lactate, degradation is very important for coaches to train athletes to see training gains. In an untrained individual, the LT can occur between 40 and 60% of VO_{2max}. However, in elite endurance athletes, the LT can occur between 70 and 85% of VO_{2max}. Understanding where the LT occurs and how to determine it is a secondary test to aerobic capacity.

How Do Different Methods of Laboratory and Field Assessments of Aerobic Capacity Compare?

Assessment of aerobic capacity can be completed in the laboratory setting or in the field. This testing can be completed as either maximal or submaximal depending upon the setting that it is taking place. Traditionally, in the laboratory setting, the protocol that is selected is a graded exercise test (GXT) which is typically considered a maximal test. The protocol consists of the individual performing the testing to volitional fatigue on a treadmill, cycle ergometer, or other device. The protocol selected could be the Bruce protocol on a treadmill or a continuous increasing workload on a cycle ergometer. In the laboratory setting, the use of a metabolic cart (Figure 10.1) monitors specific physiological variables including VO_2, volume of carbon dioxide (VCO_2), respiratory exchange ratio (RER), heart rate (HR), minute ventilation (V_E), and many others. However, field tests like the 12-minute run (Cooper 1968), 15-minute run (Balke, 1963), the Queens College step test (Mcardle et al., 1972), Astrand step test (Marley and Linnerud, 1976), or the YMCA cycle ergometer test (Golding 2000) either use an extrapolation method based upon heart rate and power output or regression model to estimate VO_{2max}.

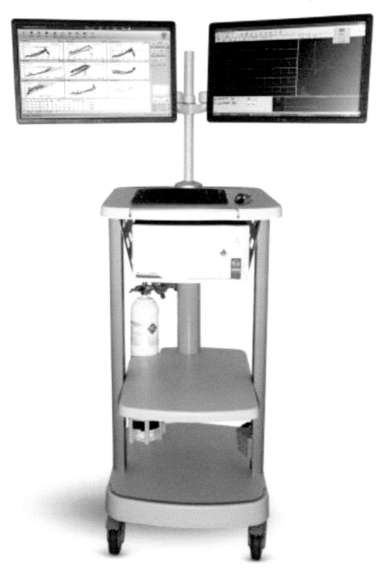

Figure 10.1 Example of COSMED Quark CPET metabolic cart.

Part 2: Maximal Exercise Testing

Maximal exercise testing enables individuals to assess cardiorespiratory capacity. When working with athletes, it is very important to select the best test possible that will maximize the individuals' training or type of sport; in addition, selecting the protocol based upon age and health and fitness status. Traditional testing is conducted on a treadmill or cycle ergometer. However, if working with athletes which are wheelchair bound or another issue that does not allow the individuals to use their legs, arm-crank ergometry can be used.

The exercise-testing protocol can be continuous or discontinuous. A continuous exercise test is performed without any rest between workload changes. Continuous exercise tests may vary in total length of time during each stage and the increase in workload from one stage to the next. Previous research has suggested that the total length of time for the test is between 8 and 12 minutes to achieve VO_{2max} (Gibbons et al., 2002; Fletcher et al., 2013). However, the timing may be less due to the less fit of an individual or longer if the individual is highly fit (Beltz et al., 2016). Consideration may be made in severely unfit individuals, but that is beyond the scope of this manual.

A continuous test is one of the most popular tests that are used in different testing laboratories. The ramp protocol provides continuous and frequent increases in work rate throughout the test so that VO_2 increases linearly.

Criteria for VO_{2max}

There have been several criteria that have been proposed for the determination of VO_{2max}. The main criterion is that VO_2 attains a plateau despite an increase in workload. This is highly debated presently. In addition, commonly used criteria are the RER value greater than or equal to 1.10, a 5-minute post-exercise blood lactate of greater than 8.0 mmol/L^{-1}, HR within plus/minus (+/−) 10 beats·min^{-1} of age-predicted maximal heart rate (APMHR), and a rate of perceived exertion (RPE) of 18 or higher (6–20 scale) on the Borg scale. The additional criteria are supplementary to the main criterion of a plateau of VO_2, and do not indicate if VO_{2max} has been achieved. It is very common for elite athletes to achieve most if not all these criteria.

Determining a plateau in VO_2 has been highly debated by several researchers (Taylor et al., 1955; Howley et al., 1995; Beltrami et al., 2012). Taylor et al. cited the plateau of VO_2 as VO_2 of less than 2.1 ml·kg^{-1}·min^{-1} or less than 150 ml·min^{-1}. Astrand (1961) described it as a levelling of VO_2 uptake. In another study, Astrand (1960) reported the plateau to occur at VO_2 of 80 ml/min^{-1}. Issekutz et al. (1969) established a plateau of less than 100 ml·min^{-1}. Cumming and Friesen reported the plateau of VO_2 as less than 50 ml·min^{-1}. Many researchers will use the criterion of VO_2 plateau of less than 150 ml·min^{-1}. However, if the criterion of a plateau in VO_2 does not happen, consider having the participant return to the lab for a follow-up test to determine if the VO_2 that was attained at peak exercise is repeatable on subsequent testing.

Graded Exercise Treadmill Test Protocol

Reason for Test

This test is used to determine VO_{2max}, velocity at VO_{2max}, LT, LTP/RCP, and economy during running. Traditionally, this test can be a continuous or discontinuous protocol depending upon how the test is selected. Prior to the test being started, a finger-tip sample of blood is taken to determine resting La$^-$. This technique of La$^-$ measurement is taken following each stage during the test and pulmonary gas exchange and heart rate data will be collected throughout as well.

Test Protocol

The test begins with an initial warm-up period of 10–15 minutes of jogging at a self-selected pace. The treadmill grade will be set at 1.0% to stimulate the energetic cost of outdoor running (Jones and Doust, 1996). Upon completion of the warm-up, the speed for the first stage will be set at 11–15 km/hr^{-1} (6.8–9.3 mi/hr^{-1}), depending upon the fitness of the athlete. The speed will be increased 1 km/hr^{-1} (0.6 mi·hr^{-1}) every 3 minutes. At the end of each stage, the athlete should straddle the treadmill belt and place their arms on the guardrails to support their body weight while the sample is being taken. The athlete will resume running once the sample is taken (~10–15 seconds). The time for the stage will start once the athlete is running again. The goal is for the athlete complete as many stages as possible with an endpoint of volitional fatigue (i.e. HR within 5–10 b/min^{-1} of maximum, blood La$^-$ > 4.0 mM). Upon completion of the test, the final speed should be noted. This is the velocity at VO$_{2max}$. Upon completion of the final stage of the test, a period of active recovery (e.g. walking or light jogging on the treadmill) is of approximately 15 minutes. To determine running economy, the treadmill speed will be placed at the speed of 2 km·hr^{-1} (1.2 mi·/hr^{-1}) below the maximal speed that was completed earlier in the test. The speed will be increased to velocity at VO$_{2max}$. Once this is achieved, the treadmill grade will be increased by 1.0% every minute until the runner can no longer tolerate (may last 5–10 minutes). Pulmonary gas exchange and heart monitoring will be continued throughout the test. Blood La$^-$ should be taken at the end of the test and during recovery from the test during minutes 1, 3, 5, 7, and 10 post-exercise.

Data Interpretation

Data from the initial portion of the treadmill test are used to determine LT, LTP/RCP, and running economy. LT and LTP/RCP are determined by plotting La$^-$ values against speed (Figure 10.2). Running economy can be expressed relative to body mass

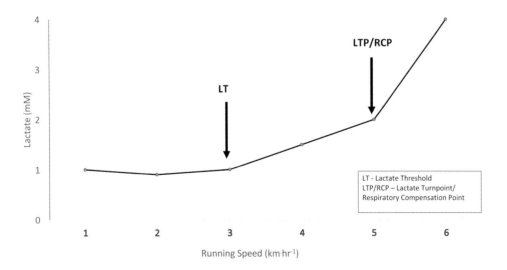

Figure 10.2 A graphic representation of blood lactate collection during the different stages of treadmill running. LT – lactate threshold; LTP/RCP – lactate turnpoint/respiratory compensation point.

Table 10.1 General classification of running economy expressed as the VO_2 cost of running a specific speed and the O_2 cost of running a specific distance.

Classification	VO_2 at 16 km/hr^{-1} (ml/kg^{-1}/min^{-1})	O_2 Cost of Running (ml/kg^{-1}/min^{-1})
Excellent	44–47	170–180
Very good	47–50	180–190
Average	50–54	190–210
Poor	55–48	210–220

for each stage as the VO_2 cost (during the last 60-seconds of the stage) of running a particular speed or a specific distance (Table 10.1).

Determination of VO_{2max} and velocity at VO_{2max} is determined during the second phase of the treadmill protocol. When determining VO_{2max} from the data collected, there is much variability when collecting VO_2 breath-by-breath, so do not determine VO_{2max} from one breath (i.e. the highest one), use the highest 30-second average during the final 20 seconds at the end of exercise and first 10 seconds of recovery. Once determined, VO_{2max} can be reported in absolute and relative (to body mass) terms and compared to normative data for athletes (Table 10.2). The velocity at VO_{2max} can be determined by multiplying the measured relative VO_{2max} by 60 and dividing the product by the running economy (in ml/kg^{-1}/min^{-1}) determined from the first part of the protocol.

Ramp Incremental Cycling Test Protocol

Reason for Test

The ramp incremental cycling test determines similar results as the treadmill test, VO_{2max}, exercise economy, ventilatory threshold (VT), and RCP. This protocol requires the use of a cycle ergometer that can increase the workload continuously. This test was initially developed by Whipp et al. (1981) and used an electronically braked ergometer to determine aerobic function.

Test Protocol

The test begins with the athlete pedalling at a predetermined cadence with a work rate set at 40–50 W to account for the mean response time to the internal O_2 cost and the internal resistance of the cycle ergometer (Boone and Bourgois, 2012). Selecting the best pedal cadence is important as too low may increase the delta (Δ) VO_2/Δ work

Table 10.2 General classifications of VO_{2max} relative to body mass (ml/kg^{-1}/min^{-1}) at a variety of levels of performance for male and female athletes.

Classification	Male	Female
World class	80–90	70–80
International	70–80	60–70
National	65–75	55–65
College-age individual	40–50	35–45

rate (Jones et al., 2004) as well as recruitment of type II muscle fibers (Beelen and Sargent, 1993; Sargent, 1994). Pulmonary gas exchange and HR data are collected throughout, and blood will be drawn at the end of each stage to determine La⁻. The test will begin after the completion of the 5-minute warm-up period. The increase in workload should be selected to complete the test within 10 minutes of volitional fatigue. The test will be completed when the athlete can no longer maintain the same pedal cadence and there is a drop in cadence of greater than 10 rev·min⁻¹ despite maximal effort. Verbal encouragement from the tester should be completed throughout the test especially at the end of the test. A form of active recovery should be completed post exercise.

Data Interpretation

Data interpretation should be very similar to the treadmill protocol. VO_{2peak} should be determined as previously discussed in the treadmill protocol, do not take the highest data point, the data should be averaged across 15 seconds or 30 seconds and the final average should be taken from the last 30 seconds of the test and first 15 seconds of active recovery.

The VT is determined by examining the relationship between VCO_2 and VO_2 responses by Beaver et al. (1986) and Whipp et al. (1981). This relationship is called the V-slope method (Figure 10.3).

Additional data that is collected via the metabolic cart includes minute ventilation (V_E), so a second analysis can be completed using the ventilatory equivalents of O_2 (V_E/VO_2) and CO_2 (V_E/VCO_2). The ventilatory equivalents are defined as the ratio of the volume of air ventilated (V_E) and the amount of O_2 consumed or CO_2 produced. When utilizing these variables, the estimated LT is defined as the point where there is a systematic increase in the V_E/VO_2 without a concomitant increase in the V_E/VCO_2. The RCP is defined as the point where there is a systematic rise in the V_E/VCO_2 with an increasing V_E/VO_2 (Figure 10.4).

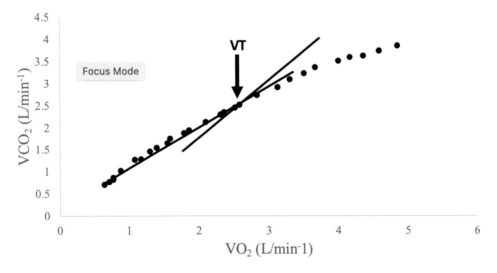

Figure 10.3 V-slope method for determination of ventilatory threshold.

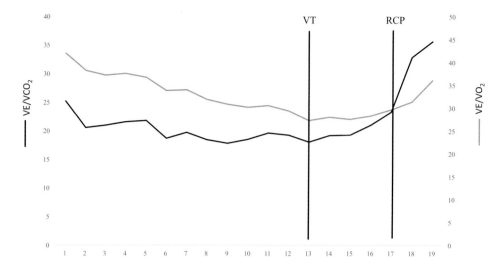

Figure 10.4 Ventilatory equivalents for oxygen and carbon dioxide. This data is from a healthy male athlete.

Field Testing

Yo-Yo Intermittent Recovery Test Levels 1 and 2.

Reason for Test

The Yo-Yo Intermittent Recovery Test (IR) tests evaluate an athlete's ability to repeatedly perform intense exercise (Bangsbo et al., 2008). The Yo-Yo IR level 1 test focuses on the aerobic system, and the Yo-Yo IR level 2 focuses on the ability to recover from repeated exercise bouts via the anaerobic system. Several sports like basketball (Castagna et al., 2008; Vernillo et al., 2012), soccer (Mohr et al., 2003; Krustrup et al., 2005), rugby (Atkins, 2006; Dobbin et al., 2018), and running (Iaia et al., 2006) have extensively used the Yo-Yo IR to evaluate athletes.

Test Protocol

The test involves having the athlete running back and forth on a field that has a defined start and finish line and turn lines or cones placed 20 m apart. This test can be performed indoors or outdoors depending on choice based upon the small space required for testing. An additional cone is placed 5 m behind the start and finish lines. The Yo-Yo IR tests consist of 2×20-m shuttle runs at increasing speeds, interspersed with a 10-second period of active recovery which is controlled by sounds from a recording. The athlete will complete the 20-m shuttle run until he is unable to maintain the speed, and distance covered the test will be ended. The Yo-Yo IR level 1 starts at a lower speed and with the increases being more moderate than the Yo-Yo IR level 2 test. The Yo-Yo IR level 1 test lasts approximately 10–20 minutes, whereas the level 2 test will be completed within 5–15 minutes. Upon completion of a warm-up, the protocol will be set at four bouts at 10.0–13.0 $km \cdot hr^{-1}$ followed by seven bouts at 13.5–14.0 km/hr^{-1} (Krustrup et al., 2003). The test will continue with increases of 0.5 $km \cdot hr^{-1}$ after every eight bouts until the test is terminated when the athlete cannot reach the finish lines two times in a row. The total distance covered prior to the test being terminated is recorded as the result.

Data Interpretation

The total distance covered can be placed into a regression equation to estimate VO_{2max} (Bangsbo et al., 2008) (Equations for Yo-Yo IR test Levels 1 and 2). The Yo-Yo IR test has been demonstrated to be a reliable measurement that can be used to examine changes in performance over time (Bangsbo et al., 2008).

$$VO_{2max} = 0.0084x + 36.4 \ (\text{Level 1})$$

$$VO_{2max} = 0.0136x + 45.3 \ (\text{Level 2})$$

Where x is the total distance covered. However, changes in performance via the Yo-Yo IR tests are considerably greater than changes in VO_{2max} and may be more accurate reflecting repeated ability during intense exercise (Bangsbo et al., 2008).

Additional Running Tests

Reason for the Test

The most used distance run tests involve distances of 1.0 or 1.5 mi (1,600 or 2,400 m) to estimate VO_{2max}. Distance runs are based upon the assumption that fitter athletes will complete the distances in a shorter time compared to a less fit individual. Disch et al. (1975) reported that distances greater than 1.0 mi (1600 m) evaluate the endurance athlete better than the speed athlete. Endurance running performance can be influenced by several factors including motivation, percent fat (Cureton et al., 1978), running efficiency, LT (Costill and Fox, 1969), and body mass.

The correlations between running distance tests and VO_{2max} vary considerably ($r^2 = 0.29 - 0.97$) depending upon the age, sex, and training status. Generally, the longer the test distance, the higher the correlation with VO_{2max}. Testing should be at least 1.0 mi (1,600 m) or of a duration of 9 minutes.

Test Protocol for the 12-minute Run Test

When performing a running distance test, it may be best to use a 400 m track or flat course with measured distances. So, the number of laps can be counted and multiplied by the distance. Markers should be placed to divide the course into quarters or eighths of a mile so that it can quickly determine the exact distance covered in a 12-minute period. At the end of the test, calculate the total distance covered in meters and use the appropriate equation to estimate the VO_{2max} (Table 10.3).

Table 10.3 Prediction equations for cardiorespiratory field tests.

Test	Equation	Source
1.0 mi steady-state jog	$VO_{2max} = 100.5 - 0.1636$ (BM, kg) $- 1.438$ (time, min) $- 0.1928$ (HR) $+ 8.344$ (gender, 1,0)	George et al. 1993
1.5 mi run/walk (women)	$VO_{2max} = 88.02 - 0.1656$ (BM, kg) $- 2.76$ (run time, min)	George et al. 1993
1.5 mi run/walk (women)	$VO_{2max} = 91.736 - 0.1656$ (BM, kg) $- 2.76$ (run time, min)	George et al. 1993
1.5 mi run/walk	$VO_{2max} = 100.16 + 7.30$ (gender, 1,0) $- 0.164$ (BM, kg) $- 1.273$ (time, min)	Larsen et al. 2002
12-min run	$VO_{2max} = 0.0268$ (distance, m) $- 11.3$	Cooper 1968
15-min run	$VO_{2max} = 0.0178$ (distance, m) $+ 9.6$	Balke 1963
1.0 mi walk	$VO_{2max} = 132.853 - 0.0769$ (BM, lb) $- 0.3877$ (age, yr) $+ 6.315$ (gender, 1,0) $- 3.2469$ (time, min) $- 0.1565$ (HR)	Kline et al. 1987

HR = heart rate; m = meters; BM = body mass; kg = kilograms; lb = pounds.
For gender substitute 1 for males and 0 for females.

Testing Protocol for the 1.0–1.5-mile Run/Walk Test

This test should be completed on a 400-m track or measured area. Consider using a measuring wheel when not completing the test on a track. The test should be completed in the fastest time possible, and walking is allowed, but the object of the test is to complete the test in the shortest period of time. Pacing is very important during this test to attain the best possible outcome. Heart rate should be monitored throughout as HR will be needed to be included in the equation to estimate VO_{2max}. Additionally, gender, body mass, and elapsed time should be recorded as well. Time will need to be converted to minutes. So, divide the seconds by 60 to calculate minutes. An example would be that a time of 15:15 exercise time is converted to 15.25 (15/60 sec = 0.25 min) (Table 10.3).

Case Study: VO₂ₘₐₓ Testing

A 40-year-old man performed a maximal cycle ergometer test to determine his VO_{2max} that was requested by his coach. He has been an avid cyclist in prior years but does not race at time of testing. He has no exercise-related symptoms and denies any chronic medical conditions. He does not take any medications and is apparently healthy. Prior to exercise, basic demographics were recorded (Table 10.4).

The participant began with 2 minutes of resting while on the cycle ergometer which was followed by 2 minutes of unloaded cycling at 60 rpm. Once unloaded cycling was completed, the workload was increased by 25 W/min^{-1} until volitional fatigue. A metabolic cart collected VO_2, VCO_2, HR, and VE throughout the exercise protocol. Once the test was terminated, 2 minutes of recovery was completed. Data is recorded in Table 10.5. Anaerobic threshold is determined in Figure 10.4.

The test demonstrates a VO_{2max} of 43.3 ml/kg^{-1}/min^{-1} for this participant. Additionally, his AT occurred at 2.49 L·min^{-1} (66.6% of VO_{2max}) (Figure 10.5). This study was well performed and would be considered maximal based upon the following criteria: plateau of VO_2 with increasing workload, HR within $\pm$ 10 b·min^{-1} of

Table 10.4 Men's and women's aerobic fitness classifications based upon age and relative VO_2.

Category	Men 13–19	20–29	Age (years) 30–39	40–49	50–59	60+
Very Poor	< 35.0	< 33.0	< 31.5	< 30.2	< 26.1	< 20.5
Poor	35.0–38.3	33.0–36.4	31.5–35.4	30.2–33.5	26.1–30.9	20.5–26.0
Fair	38.4–45.1	36.5–42.4	35.5–40.9	33.6–38.9	31.0–35.7	26.1–32.2
Good	45.2–50.9	42.5–46.4	41.0–44.9	39.0–43.7	35.8–40.9	32.3–36.4
Excellent	51.0–55.9	46.5–52.5	45.0–49.4	43.8–48.0	41.0–45.3	36.5–44.2
Superior	> 56.0	> 52.5	> 49.5	> 48.1	> 45.4	> 44.3

All values of VO_{2max} are in $ml \cdot kg^{-1} \cdot min^{-1}$ (Cooper, 1977)

Category	Women 13-19	20–29	Age (years) 30–39	40–49	50–59	60+
Very Poor	< 25.0	< 23.6	< 22.8	< 21.0	< 20.2	< 17.5
Poor	25.0–30.9	23.6–28.9	22.8–26.9	21.0–24.4	20.2–22.7	17.5–20.1
Fair	31.0–34.9	29.0–32.9	27.0–31.4	24.5–28.9	22.8–26.9	20.2–24.4
Good	35.0–38.9	33.0–36.9	31.5–35.6	29.0–32.8	27.0–31.4	24.5–30.2
Excellent	39.0–41.9	37.0–40.9	35.7–40.0	32.9–36.9	31.5–35.7	30.3–31.4
Superior	> 42.0	> 41.0	> 40.1	> 37.0	> 35.8	> 31.5

All values of VO_{2max} are in $ml \cdot kg^{-1} \cdot min^{-1}$ (Cooper, 1977)

Table 10.5 Data collection for a case study.

Time (min)	Workload (W)	HR (bpm)	VE (L/min)	VO_2 (L/min)	VCO_2 (L/min)	RER	VE/VCO_2	VE/VO_2
1	Rest	53	10.4	0.33	0.31	0.93	34	32
2	Rest	64	11.3	0.44	0.37	0.84	31	26
3	Unloaded	77	19.9	0.76	0.67	0.88	30	26
4	Unloaded	82	21.0	0.78	0.70	0.89	30	27
5	25	86	22.6	0.83	0.77	0.93	29	27
6	50	90	23.8	1.02	0.88	0.86	27	23
7	75	101	31.8	1.29	1.17	0.91	27	25
8	100	106	35.7	1.55	1.40	0.90	26	23
9	125	115	39.2	1.76	1.59	0.90	25	22
10	150	120	44.9	1.94	1.86	0.96	24	23
11	175	132	56.4	2.30	2.31	1.01	24	25
12	200	138	59.2	2.46	2.52	1.03	23	24
13	225	146	61.8	2.74	2.83	1.04	22	23
14	250	152	74.0	3.09	3.30	1.07	22	24
15	275	162	80.9	3.36	3.67	1.09	22	24
16	300	168	94.3	3.59	4.17	1.16	23	26
17	325	172	108.8	3.74	4.59	1.23	24	29
18	Recovery	159	84.2	2.05	3.36	1.63	25	41
19	Recovery	131	57.9	1.30	2.01	1.54	29	45

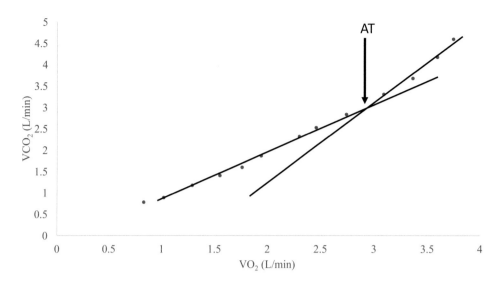

Figure 10.5 Anaerobic threshold determination using V-Slope method for case study.

age-predicted maximum HR, and RER > 1.15. Based upon Table 10.4, this participant aerobic fitness would be classified in the Excellent category.

Laboratory Task: How "Fit" Are You?

Complete a VO_{2max} test and determine the different thresholds based upon the test. If possible, complete a test on a treadmill and cycle ergometer and compare the tests. Are the results similar or different and why? Review the results and compare results to normative data.

Lab Results for Treadmill Test

Subject Name _____   Gender _____   Age (y) _____

Height (cm) _____   Weight (kg) _____   BMI (kg/m²) _____

Room Temp (C) _____ P_B (mmHg) _____   Humidity (&) _____

Stage	Time	Speed (mph)	Grade (%)	VO_2 ($L \cdot min^{-1}$)	VCO_2 ($L \cdot min^{-1}$)	RER	BLa-

Absolute VO_{2max} ($L \cdot min^{-1}$) _____   Relative VO_{2max} ($ml \cdot kg \cdot min^{-1}$) _____

Classification _____

Graph to draw LT, VT, and RCP.

Evaluation/Comments:

_____

_____

_____

_____

Lab Results for Cycle Ergometer Test

Subject Name _____   Gender _____   Age (y) _____

Height (cm) _____   Weight (kg) _____   BMI (kg/m²) _____

Room Temp. (C) _____ P_B (mmHg) _____   Humidity (&) _____

Stage	Time	Cadence (rpm)	Resistance (W)	VO₂ (L·min⁻¹)	VCO₂ (L·min⁻¹)	RER	BLa-

Absolute VO_{2max} (L·min⁻¹) _____   Relative VO_{2max} (ml·kg·min⁻¹) _____

Classification _____

Graph to draw LT, VT, and RCP.

Evaluation/Comments:

_____

_____

_____

_____

Yo-Yo Intermittent Recovery Test Level 1

Name: _____   Gender: _____

Sport: _____   Age (years): _____

Body Mass (kg): _____   Height (cm): _____

Level	Speed Level	Shuttles (2 × 20m)	Speed (km·hr⁻¹)	Accumulated Distance (m)	Completed (Y/N)
1	5	1	10.0	40	
2	9	1	12.0	80	
3	11	1	13.0	120	
4	11	2	13.5	160	
5	12	1	13.5	200	
6	12	2	13.5	240	
7	12	3	13.5	280	
8	13	1	14.0	320	
9	13	2	14.0	360	
10	13	3	14.0	400	
11	13	4	14.0	440	
12	14	1	14.0	480	
13	14	2	14.0	520	
14	14	3	14.5	560	
15	14	4	14.5	600	
16	14	5	14.5	640	
17	14	6	14.5	680	
18	14	7	14.5	720	
19	14	8	14.5	760	
20	15	1	15.0	800	
21	15	2	15.0	840	
22	15	3	15.0	880	
23	15	4	15.0	920	
24	15	5	15.0	960	
25	15	6	15.0	1000	
26	15	7	15.0	1040	
27	15	8	15.0	1080	
28	16	1	15.5	1120	
29	16	2	15.5	1160	
30	16	3	15.5	1200	
31	16	4	15.5	1240	
32	16	5	15.5	1280	
33	16	6	15.5	1320	
34	16	7	15.5	1360	
35	16	8	15.5	1400	
36	17	1	16.0	1440	

(Continued)

Level	Speed Level	Shuttles (2 × 20m)	Speed (km·hr⁻¹)	Accumulated Distance (m)	Completed (Y/N)
37	17	2	16.0	1480	
38	17	3	16.0	1520	
39	17	4	16.0	1560	
40	17	5	16.0	1600	
41	17	6	16.0	1640	
42	17	7	16.0	1680	
43	17	8	16.0	1720	
44	18	1	16.5	1760	
45	18	2	16.5	1800	
46	18	3	16.5	1840	
47	18	4	16.5	1880	
48	18	5	16.5	1920	
49	18	6	16.5	1960	
50	18	7	16.5	2000	
51	18	8	16.5	2040	
52	19	1	17.0	2080	
53	19	2	17.0	2120	
54	19	3	17.0	2160	
55	19	4	17.0	2200	
56	19	5	17.0	2240	
57	19	6	17.0	2280	
58	19	7	17.0	2320	
59	19	8	17.0	2360	
60	20	1	17.5	2400	
61	20	2	17.5	2440	
62	20	3	17.5	2480	
63	20	4	17.5	2520	
64	20	5	17.5	2560	
65	20	6	17.5	2600	
66	20	7	17.5	2640	
67	21	8	17.5	2680	
68	21	1	18.0	2720	
69	21	2	18.0	2760	
70	21	3	18.0	2800	
71	21	4	18.0	2840	
72	21	5	18.0	2880	
73	21	6	18.0	2920	
74	21	7	18.0	2960	
75	21	8	18.0	3000	
76	22	1	18.5	3040	
77	22	2	18.5	3080	

(Continued)

Level	Speed Level	Shuttles (2 × 20m)	Speed (km·hr⁻¹)	Accumulated Distance (m)	Completed (Y/N)
78	22	3	18.5	3120	
79	22	4	18.5	3160	
80	22	5	18.5	3200	
81	22	6	18.5	3240	
82	22	7	18.5	3280	
83	22	8	18.5	3320	
84	23	1	19.0	3360	
85	23	2	19.0	3400	
86	23	3	19.0	3440	
87	23	4	19.0	3480	
88	23	5	19.0	3520	
89	23	6	19.0	3560	
90	23	7	19.0	3600	
91	23	8	19.0	3640	

Bangsbo et al. (2008)

Calculate $VO_{2max} = 0.0084x + 36.4$

VO_{2max} = _____

Evaluation/Comments:

_____
_____
_____
_____

Yo-Yo Intermittent Recovery Test Level 2

Name: _____   Gender: _____

Sport: _____   Age (years): _____

Body Mass (kg): _____   Height (cm): _____

Level	Speed Level	Shuttles (2 × 20 m)	Speed (km·hr⁻¹)	Accumulated Distance (m)	Completed (Y/N)
1	11	1	13.0	40	
2	15	1	15.0	80	
3	17	1	16.0	120	
4	17	2	16.0	160	
5	18	1	16.5	200	
6	18	2	16.5	240	
7	18	3	16.5	280	
8	19	1	17.0	320	
9	19	2	17.0	360	
10	19	3	17.0	400	
11	19	4	17.0	440	
12	20	1	17.5	480	
13	20	2	17.5	520	
14	20	3	17.5	560	
15	20	4	17.5	600	
16	20	5	17.5	640	
17	20	6	17.5	680	
18	20	7	17.5	720	
19	20	8	17.5	760	
20	21	1	18.0	800	
21	21	2	18.0	840	
22	21	3	18.0	880	
23	21	4	18.0	920	
24	21	5	18.0	960	
25	21	6	18.0	1000	
26	21	7	18.0	1040	
27	21	8	18.0	1080	
28	22	1	18.5	1120	
29	22	2	18.5	1160	
30	22	3	18.5	1200	
31	22	4	18.5	1240	
32	22	5	18.5	1280	
33	22	6	18.5	1320	
34	22	7	18.5	1360	
35	22	8	18.5	1400	
36	23	1	19.0	1440	
37	23	2	19.0	1480	
38	23	3	19.0	1520	
39	23	4	19.0	1560	
40	23	5	19.0	1600	
41	23	6	19.0	1640	
42	23	7	19.0	1680	
43	23	8	19.0	1720	
44	24	1	19.5	1760	
45	24	2	19.5	1800	
46	24	3	19.5	1840	

(Continued)

Level	Speed Level	Shuttles (2 × 20 m)	Speed (km·hr⁻¹)	Accumulated Distance (m)	Completed (Y/N)
47	24	4	19.5	1880	
48	24	5	19.5	1920	
49	24	6	19.5	1960	
50	24	7	19.5	2000	
51	24	8	19.5	2040	
52	25	1	20.0	2080	
53	25	2	20.0	2120	
54	25	3	20.0	2160	
55	25	4	20.0	2200	
56	25	5	20.0	2240	
57	25	6	20.0	2280	
58	25	7	20.0	2320	
59	25	8	20.0	2360	
60	26	1	20.5	2400	
61	26	2	20.5	2440	
62	26	3	20.5	2480	
63	26	4	20.5	2520	
64	26	5	20.5	2560	
65	26	6	20.5	2600	
66	26	7	20.5	2640	
67	26	8	20.5	2680	

(Bangsbo et al., 2008)

Calculate $VO_{2max} = 0.0136x + 45.3$

$VO_{2max} =$ _____

Evaluation/Comments:

_____
_____
_____
_____

Aerobic Capacity Test - 1.5-mile run Data and Calculation

Name: _____   Gender: _____

Sport: _____   Age (years): _____

Body Mass (kg): _____   Height (cm): _____

1.5-mile run time (minutes): _____

Calculate the athlete's estimated VO_{2max} from the 1.5-mile run test.

Female athlete: $VO_{2max} = 88.02 - 0.1656 \text{ (BM, kg)} - 2.76 \text{ (run time, min)}$

$VO_{2max} =$ _____

Male athlete = $VO_{2max} = 91.736 - 0.1656 \text{ (BM, kg)} - 2.76 \text{ (run time, min)}$

$VO_{2max} =$ _____

Classification of athlete's estimated VO_{2max} from the 1.5-mile run test (Table 10.3).

Classification: _____

Evaluation/Comments:

_____

_____

_____

_____

Aerobic Capacity Test - 12-minunte run test Data Collection and Calculation

Name: _____   Gender: _____

Sport: _____   Age (years): _____

Body Mass (kg): _____   Height (cm): _____

12-minute run distance (m): _____

Calculate the athlete's estimated VO_{2max} from the 12-minute run test.

$VO_{2max} = 0.0268$ (distance, m) $- 11.3$

$VO_{2max} =$ _____

Classification of athlete's estimated VO_{2max} from the 12-minute run test (Table 10.3).

Classification: _____

Evaluation/Comments:

_____

_____

_____

_____

Summary

The purpose of this chapter has been to present the reasons for methods, and the types of testing to measure aerobic capacity in athletes. While measuring the aerobic capacity of an athlete requires there to be an understanding that while measuring maximal oxygen consumption, there is an anaerobic component to the testing which may entail understanding all abilities of the athlete. Thus, the characteristics of performance require an understanding of different concepts including the LT as well as the integration of the anaerobic testing incorporated into the testing helps evaluate the complete measurement of aerobic capacity.

The literature has demonstrated that maximal oxygen consumption may demonstrate the functional capacity, but certainly does not demonstrate the abilities of the athlete. Although a cyclist may have a VO_{2max} of 84 ml/kg^{-1}/min^{-1} does not mean that they will be able to win the Tour de France. However, understanding what the values that are measured gives a snapshot and can be incorporated into their training program. In addition, establishing the proper testing protocol and criteria needs to be set prior to testing and should be individualized for the athlete.

References

ACSM. 2021. *ACSM's Guidelines for Exercise Testing and Prescription*, 11th ed. Philadelphia, PA: Wouters Kluwer.

Astrand, I. 1960. Aerobic work capacity in men and women with special reference to age. *Acta Physiol Scand*, 49, 1–92.

Atkins, S. J. 2006. Performance of the Yo-Yo intermittent recovery test by elite professional and semiprofessional Rugby league players. *J Strength Cond Res*, 20, 222–5.

Balke, B. 1963. A simple field test for the assessment of physical fitness.. REP 63-6. [Report]. Civil Aeromedical Research Institute (U.S.), 1–8.

Bangsbo, J., Iaia, F. M. & Krustrup, P. 2008. The Yo-Yo intermittent recovery test: A useful tool for evaluation of physical performance in intermittent sports. *Sports Med*, 38, 37–51.

Beaver, W. L., Wasserman, K. & Whipp, B. J. 1986. A new method for detecting anaerobic threshold by gas exchange. *J Appl Physiol*, 60, 2020–7.

Beelen, A. & Sargent, A. J. 1993. Effect of prior exercise at different pedalling frequencies on maximal power in humans. *Euro J Appl Physiol*, 66, 102–7.

Beltrami, F. G., Froyd, C., Mauger, A. R., Metcalfe, A. J., Marino, F. & Noakes, T. D. 2012. Conventional testing methods produce submaximal values of maximum oxygen consumption. *Br J Sports Med*, 46, 23–29.

Beltz, N. M., Gibson, A. L., Janot, J. M., Kravitz, L., Mermier, C. M., & Dalleck, L. C. (2016). Graded Exercise Testing Protocols for the Determination of VO_2max: Historical Perspectives, Progress, and Future Considerations. *J Sports Med (Hindawi Publ Corp)*, 2016, 3968393.

Beneke, R., Leithauser, R. M. & Ochentel, O. 2011. Blood lactate diagnostics in exercise testing and training. *Int J Sports Physiol Perform*, 6, 8–24.

Billat, V. L., Sirvent, P., Py, G., Horalsztein, J. P. & Mercier, J. 2003. The concept of maximal lactate steady state: A bridge between biochemistry, physiology and sport science. *Sports Med*, 33, 407–26.

Boone, J. & Bourgois, J. 2012. The oxygen uptake response to incremental ramp exercise: Methodological and physiological issues. *Sports Med*, 42, 511–26.

Castagna, C., Imperllizzeri, F. M., Rampinini, E., D'ottavio, S. & Manzi, V. 2008. The Yo-Yo intermittent recovery test in basketball players. *J Sci Med Sport*, 11, 202–8.

Cooper, K. H. 1968. A means of assessing maximal oxygen uptake. *JAMA*, 203, 201–4.

Costill, D. C. & Fox, E. L. 1969. Energetics of marathon running. *Med Sci Sports*, 1, 81–6.

Cumming, G. R. & Friesen, W. 1969. Bicycle ergometer measurement of maximal oxygen uptake in children. *Can J Pharmacol*, 45, 937–46.

Cureton, K. J., Sparling, P. B., Evans, B. W., Johnson, S. M., Kong, U. D. & Purvis, J. W. 1978. Effect of experimental alterations in excess weight on aerobic capacity and distance running performance. *Med Scie Sports*, 10, 194–9.

Davis, H. A., Bassett, J., Hughes, P. & Gass, G. C. 1983. Anaerobic threshold and lactate turnpoint. *Euro J Appl Physiol*, 50, 383–92.

Davis, H. A. & Gass, G. C. 1979. Blood lactate concentrations during incremental work before and after maximum exercise. *Br J Sports Med*, 13, 165–9.

Disch, J., Frankiewicz, R. & Jackson, A. 1975. Construct validation of distance run tests. *Res Quart*, 46, 169–76.

Dobbin, N., Moss, S. L., Highton, J. & Twist, C. 2018. An examination of a modified YO-YO to measure intermittent running performance in Rugby players. *Eur J Sport Sci*, 18, 1068–76.

Farrell, P. A., Wilmore, J. H., Coyle, E. F., Billing, J. E. & Costill, D. L. 1979. Plasma lactate accumulation and distance running performance. *Med Sci Sports Exer*, 11, 338–44.

Fletcher, G. F., Ades, P. A., Kligfield, P., Arena, R., Balady, G. J., Bittner, V. A., Coke, L. A., Fleg, J. L., Forman, D. E., Gerber, T. C., Gulati, M., Madan, K., Rhodes, J., Thompson, P. D., Williams, M. A., & American Heart Association Exercise, Cardiac Rehabilitation, and Prevention Committee of the Council on Clinical Cardiology, Council on Nutrition, Physical Activity and Metabolism, Council on Cardiovascular and Stroke Nursing, and Council on Epidemiology and Prevention (2013). Exercise standards for testing and training: a scientific statement from the American Heart Association. *Circulation*, 128, 873–934.

George, J., Vehrs, P., Allsen, P., Fellingham, G. & Fisher, G. 1993. VO_2 max estimation from a submaximal 1-mile track jog for fit college-age individuals. *Med Sci Sports Exer*, 25, 401–6.

Gibbons, R. J., Balady, G. J., Bricker, J. T., Chaitman, B. R., Fletcher, G. F., Froelicher, V. F., Mark, D. B., McCallister, B. D., Mooss, A. N., O'Reilly, M. G., Winters, W. L., Gibbons, R. J., Antman, E. M., Alpert, J. S., Faxon, D. P., Fuster, V., Gregoratos, G., Hiratzka, L. F., Jacobs, A. K., Russell, R. O., ... American College of Cardiology/American Heart

Association Task Force on Practice Guidelines. Committee to Update the 1997 Exercise Testing Guidelines (2002). ACC/AHA 2002 guideline update for exercise testing: summary article. A report of the American College of Cardiology/American Heart Association Task Force on Practice Guidelines (Committee to Update the 1997 Exercise Testing Guidelines). *J Amer Coll Cardiol*, 40, 1531–40.

Golding, L. 2000. *The Y's Way to Physical Fitness*. Champaign, IL: Human Kinetics.

Hill, A. V., Long, C. N. H. & Lupton, H. 1924. Muscular exercise, lactic acid and the supply and utilization of oxygen. *Proc Royal Soc B*, 97, 84–138.

Hill, A. V. & Lupton, H. 1923. Muscular exercise, lactic acid and the supply and utilization of oxygen. *Quart J Med*, 16, 135–71.

Howley, E. T., Bassett, D. R. & Welch, H. 1995. Criteria for maximal oxygen uptake: Review and commentary. *Med Sci Sport Exer*, 27, 1292–301.

Iaia, F.M., Kolding, H., Gunnarsson, T., Wendell, Rostgaard, T. Nybo, L., Krustrup, P., & Bangsbo, J. 2006. Change to anaerobic training improves running economy and high intensity exercise performance in endurance runners [abstract]. In: Hoppeler, H., Reilly, T., Tsolakidid, E., et al. (eds). *11th Annual Congress of the European College of Sport Science*, 2006 Jul 5–8; Lusanne. Cologne: Sportverlag Strauss, 212–3.

Issekutz, B. Jr, Birkhead, N. C. & Rodahl, K. 1962. Use of respiratory quotients in assessment of aerobic work capcity. *J Appl Physiol*, 17, 47–50.

Jones, A. M., Campbell, I. T. & Pringle, J. S. 2004. Influence of muscle fiber type and pedal rate on the VO_2-work rate slope during ramp exercise. *Eur J Appl Physiol*, 91, 238–45.

Jones, A. M., Vanhatalo, A., Burnley, M., Morton, R. H. & Poole, D. C. 2010. Critical power: Implications for the determination of VO2max and exercise tolerance. *Med Sci Sports Exer*, 42, 1876–90.

Jones, A. M. & Doust, J. H. 1996. A 1% treadmill grade most accurately reflects the energetic cost of outdoor running. *J Sports Sci*, 14, 321–7.

Kline, G. M., Porcori, J. P., Hintermeister, R., Freedson, P. S., Ward, A., Mccarron, R. F., Ross, J. & Rippe, J. M. 1987. Estimation of VO_2 max from a one-mile track walk, gender, age, and body weight. *Med Sci Sports Exer*, 19, 253–9.

Krustrup, P., Mohr, M., Amstrup, T., Rysgaard, T., Johansen, J., Steensberg, A., Pedersen, P. K. & Bangsbo, J. 2003. The Yo-Yo intermittent recovery test: Physiological response, reliability, and validity. *Med Sci Sports Exerc*, 35, 697–705.

Krustrup, P., Mohr, M., Ellingsgaard, H. & Bangsbo, J. 2005. Physical demands during an elite female game: Importance of training status. *Med Sci Sports Exerc*, 37, 1242–8.

Larsen, G. E., George, J. D., Alexander, J. L., Fellingham, G. W., Aldana, S. R. & Parcell, A. C. 2002. Prediction of maximum oxygen consumption from walking, jogging, or running. *Res Quart Exer Sport*, 73, 66–72.

Marley, W. & Linnerud, A. 1976. A three-year study of the astrand-rhyming step test. *Res Quart*, 47, 211–7.

Mcardle, W. D., Katch, F. I., Pechar, G. S., Jacobson, L. & Ruck, S. 1972. Reliability and interrelationships between maximal oxygen intake, physical working capacity and step-test scores in college women. *Med Sci Sports*, 4, 182–6.

Mohr, M., Krustrup, P. & Bangsbo, J. 2003. Match performance of high standard soccer players with special reference to development of fatigue. *J Sport Sci*, 21, 519–28.

Sargent, A. J. 1994. Human power output and muscle fatigue. *Int J Sports Med*, 15, 116–21.

Spencer, M. R. & Gastin, P. B. 2001. Energy system contribution during 200- to 1500-m running in highly trained athletes. *Med Sci Sports Exerc*, 33, 157–62.

Tanaka, K., Matsuura, Y., Kumagai, S., Matsuzaka, A., Hirakoba, K. & Asano, K. 1983. Relationship of anaerobic threshold and onset of blood lactate accumulation with endurance performance. *Eur J Appl Physiol*, 51, –6.

Taylor, H. L., Buskirk, E. & Henschel, A. 1955. Maximal oxygen intake as an objective measure of cardio-respiratory performance. *J Appl Physiol*, 8, 73–80.

Vernillo, G., Silvestri, A. & Torre, L. A. 2012. The Yo-Yo intermittent recovery test in junior basketball players according to performance level and age group. *J Strength Cond Res*, 26, 2490–4.

Wasserman, K. & McIlroy, M. B. 1964. Detecting the threshold of anaerobic metabolism in cardiac patients during exercise. *Am J Cardiol*, 14, 844–52.

Whipp, B. J., Davis, J. A., Torres, F. & Wasserman, K. 1981. A test to determine parameters of aerobic function during exercise. *J Appl Physiol*, 50, 217–21.

Whipp, B. J., Davis, J. A. & Wasserman, K. 1989. Ventilatory control of the 'isocapnic buffering' region in rapidly-incremental exercise. *Repair Physiol*, 76, 357–67.

11 Speed

John McMahon and Paul Comfort

Part 1: Background

Introduction

Speed, particularly during running, is a fundamental component of most professional sports. Thus, the assessment of an athlete's maximal running speed (referred to henceforth as maximal sprint performance) is a common requirement of the strength and conditioning coach. Maximal sprint performance is highly regarded as an important determinant of performance in many sports, but the distance(s) over which maximal sprint performance should be assessed will depend on the typical sprint distances covered during competitive sport play and preferably, position-specific sprint distances should be considered. For example, all batters in cricket will run precisely 17.68 m between the two wickets to accumulate runs. Thus, there would be little benefit in assessing the maximal sprint performance of crickets much beyond this distance, with linear 20-m sprint assessments often chosen for this cohort (Carr et al., 2015; Foden et al., 2015; Carr et al., 2017). Also, sprinting does not occur singularly in a linear direction during competition. Results of a recent study showed that curvilinear sprinting can be reliably assessed but it is poorly related to linear sprinting (Fílter et al., 2020). Thus, they may be considered independent of one another and so assessed separately if deemed important to the sport. A standard curvilinear sprint test comprised of a 17-m distance with a 9.15-m radius distance seems to be broadly applied in both men's and women's soccer (Fílter et al., 2020; Filter et al., 2020; Kobal et al., 2021).

Fitness testing at the beginning of the pre-season training cycle is commonplace in most sports and can inform how much the athletes' fitness has been compromised during the preceding off-season period and thus identify immediate pre-season training priorities. However, it has been suggested that it may be prudent to exclude maximal-intensity fitness tests, such as maximal sprint testing, from the very early pre-season training cycle to avoid unnecessary exposure to risk of injury after a period of inactivity (clearly this will depend on what the athletes have been doing during the off-season). Identifying an appropriate window of opportunity for assessing maximal sprint performance further into the athletes' training cycle may be preferable but would be team- and context-dependent (Buchheit and Brown, 2020). Thus, the strength and conditioning coach should exercise caution when deciding upon the precise timing of any maximal sprint testing within their athletes' season(s).

Speed is usually measured as distance divided by time, but it can also be measured as stride length multiplied by stride frequency, although this is not as frequently

DOI: 10.4324/9781003186762-11

done. The Système International (SI) unit for speed is metres per second (m/s). Speed is a scalar quantity meaning that it is not prescribed a specific direction over which it is measured. Velocity, which is sometimes used interchangeably with speed, is a vector quantity which means that it has both a magnitude and a direction. Velocity is calculated as displacement divided by time. The SI unit for velocity is also metres per second (m/s). Thus, velocity can be thought of as speed in a specific direction but when just one direction is included in a speed assessment, such as when a linear sprint running test is completed, it will be identical in number to velocity. For example, if an athlete sprints forwards over 20 m in 3 seconds, their speed and velocity will both be 6.7 m/s (i.e., 20 [distance and displacement] divided by 3 [time] when rounded to one decimal place). Therefore, to measure an athlete's speed or velocity, a device that can measure both distance (or displacement) and time, or just the latter if the sprint distance is physically marked out by the tester, is usually required, or one that can allow measurement of stride length and stride frequency.

Part 2: Assessing Speed

Fully automatic timing systems, such as those used at international athletics events, are the gold standard equipment for measuring linear sprint speed (Haugen et al., 2012; Haugen and Buchheit, 2016). These systems are, however, very expensive and therefore inaccessible to most strength and conditioning coaches (Haugen and Buchheit, 2016). Thus, several alternative devices of varying practicality and precision have been proposed in the scientific literature such as stopwatches, electronic timing gates (ETGs), lasers or radars, and high-speed videography (Haugen and Buchheit, 2016). As described in Chapter 4, the strength and conditioning coach may wish to determine the concurrent validity of the sprint assessment device themselves if they are using a system which has not been validated in a peer-reviewed study.

Stopwatch

The cheapest way to assess speed is to use a simple hand-held stopwatch in conjunction with a specific test distance marked out clearly for the athlete(s). Although stopwatches are not used in professional and elite sports as much as they used to be, they are still included in speed assessments involving collegiate- and amateur-level athletes (Munshi et al., 2022; Zaragoza et al., 2022). Results of a previous study highlighted that stopwatch estimates of linear sprint times measured for a 40-yard dash were significantly shorter (i.e., faster speed) than those obtained via electronic timing (Mann et al., 2015), but were equally reliable. This study suggests that devices for quantifying sprint times should not be used interchangeably but using a single device, including the stopwatch, can yield reliable results and so track sprint performance changes over time.

Electronic Timing Gates

ETGs are commonly utilized as part of athlete fitness testing batteries (Earp and Newton, 2012) in order to provide a record of sprint times over various known distances. The majority of ETGs work via either one (single-photocell) or two (dual-photocell) infrared beam(s) being emitted to a corresponding reflector positioned directly opposite which reflects the beam(s) back to the photocell where it is detected (Yeadon et al., 1999). If multiple sets of ETGs are positioned at incremental distances along a runway, then athletes' average speed can be determined between any two beams due to a hand-held computer logging the time period between successive beam interruptions caused by the athlete passing through them (Yeadon et al., 1999). When calculating whole body (centre of mass) speed with ETGs, it is important to ensure that they are set at a height which maximizes the chances of the beams being broken by the same part of the athlete's body, which appears to be best achieved when they are set at approximately hip height (Yeadon et al., 1999). Although dual-photocell ETGs have been shown to reduce the likelihood of an athlete's arms or legs breaking the beams when compared to single-photocell ETGs (Earp and Newton, 2012; Haugen et al., 2014), the latter are still commonly used in both research and applied settings (Carr et al., 2015, Dos'Santos et al., 2017), possibly due to them being cheaper to purchase (Earp and Newton, 2012), and they have been validated against the industry gold standard used at international athletics events (Haugen et al., 2012).

Athletes' short sprint performances (typically over 5–40 m) are commonly assessed via single-photocell ETGs to monitor changes in response to training and are regularly reported within the literature across a range of sports (Carr et al., 2015; Dos'Santos et al., 2017). Despite single-photocell ETGs being capable of yielding valid sprint times (Haugen et al., 2012), it is also important that such sprint times attained by a given population are reliable and the associated measurement error is determined to allow any observed changes in sprint performance following specific training interventions to be interpreted as meaningful (Haugen and Buchheit, 2016). This can be achieved by calculating the smallest detectible difference (SDD) which, by accounting for both test-retest reliability and measurement error, provides a threshold for the minimum difference in a test score that is reflective of a real change in performance (Beckerman et al., 2001). For example, SDD values of 5.8%, 3.0%, and 2.7% have been reported for 5-, 10-, and 20 m sprint times, respectively, attained by male cricketers via single-photocell ETGs (Carr et al., 2015). More recently, SDD values of 6.1%, 4.7%, and 3.3% for men's and 3.0%, 4.0%, and 6.8% for women's maximal sprint times over 5-, 10-, and 20 m, respectively, were reported (Ripley et al., 2020). These men and women were recreationally trained, rather than high-level athletes but nevertheless, the results of the study illustrate that sprint times measured via single-photocell ETGs are sensitive enough to detect reasonably small changes, even at the amateur level (Ripley et al., 2020).

To get the most accurate static-start (most common) sprint times possible from ETGs, the strength and conditioning coach should get the athletes to begin behind the first ETG (set at the zero [i.e., start] distance) to avoid athletes accidentally triggering the first beam before commencing their maximal sprint effort. Authors of a previous study suggest starting 0.3 m behind the first ETG, as this allows the athlete to be close enough to the first ETG without accidentally triggering it whilst preventing it from becoming a flying sprint start (Altmann et al., 2015). The athletes should adopt a two-point athletic (split-leg) stance and avoid rocking backwards or taking a false step backwards before commencing the sprint test (Johnson et al., 2010). This is because different sprint start techniques yield different sprint times and so they cannot be used interchangeably (Duthie et al., 2006). Specifically, a false backward step, a crouch, and a block start were shown to produce faster sprint performances than a standing start (Salo and Bezodis, 2004; Duthie et al., 2006; Cronin et al., 2007; Frost et al., 2008; Johnson et al., 2010; Frost and Cronin, 2011), but the latter is easier to standardise and is more familiar among most athletes.

Lasers and Radars

Laser and radar devices work in a similar way to one another. Each of them is placed directly behind the athlete being tested (usually around 3–10 m behind the sprint start line) at approximately hip height, like the ETGs, to track their approximate centre of mass location (Baena-Raya et al., 2021; Ghigiarelli et al., 2022). These devices usually sample instantaneous velocity (i.e., speed with direction) data at somewhere between 50 and 100 Hz (Ashton and Jones, 2019; Baena-Raya et al., 2021), meaning they provide a more complete speed profile of the athlete than the previously mentioned devices do. Specifically, radar and laser devices illustrate more precisely when and how peak velocity (i.e., the acceleration profile) occurred within the tested sprint distance. However, they have been suggested to be most useful for the assessment of the mid-acceleration and maximum velocity phases of sprinting (i.e., at 10 m and beyond) but not the initial acceleration phase (i.e., the initial 5 m or so) due to larger biases compared with high-speed videography, which was considered to be the criterion device (Bezodis et al., 2012). Another limitation of radar and laser devices is that they are limited to linear speed assessments only, unlike ETGs which may also be utilised for curvilinear sprint tests (Fílter et al., 2020; Kobal et al., 2021).

High-Speed Videography

In the absence of access to fully automatic timing systems (Haugen and Buchheit, 2016), high-speed videography may be considered the gold standard method for measuring sprint speed (Bezodis et al., 2012; Healy et al., 2019). Although standalone high-speed video cameras (200 Hz) have been used in studies such as Bezodis et al. (2012), most currently available smartphones include a high-speed video camera capable of sampling at up to 240 Hz and have also been used successfully to quantify linear sprint running performance (Romero-Franco et al., 2017). Thus, quantifying linear sprint performance via the high-speed video incorporated into a smartphone is likely to be the most widely accessible method for the strength and conditioning coach. When using high-speed videography to quantify sprint times or speed, it is important to follow the following general guidance. First, the camera (this term will cover both standalone and phone-embedded cameras from this point on) needs to be static. Thus, a tripod is often needed to keep the camera in a fixed position. The camera needs to be positioned in the sagittal plane (side view) and at a distance that allows a sufficient view of the athlete performing the sprint. The precise distance will depend on how much of the sprint needs to be captured, but it also needs to be close enough to the athlete for their approximate centre of mass position (or the moment each foot contacts and leaves the ground, if aiming to quantify stride length and stride frequency) to be identified. If there is a requirement to measure distances (such as sprint distances or stride lengths) from the video footage, then a calibration must be performed. This occurs in the post-processing stage via whichever software is being used but will require a physical item of known dimensions (e.g., a plyometric box or a calibration frame) to be placed where the athlete will perform the sprints (i.e., along the same line of direction in which the athlete will run) and recorded by the camera once it is placed in the required position for videoing. Once a single short video of the physical item to be used for calibration purposes has been recorded, it should be removed. So long as the camera remains in the same place during the sprint testing session, there is no need to record further videos of the physical item to be used for calibration purposes. If the camera is moved, whether accidentally or intentionally, a further video of the physical item to be used for calibration purposes should be recorded so that each individual sprint video is able to be calibrated.

Part 3: Practical Examples

Task 1: Calculating Sprint Speed

Sprint times at 10-m intervals throughout the entire men's 100-m sprint race were extracted from multiple major athletic competitions (comprised of the Olympic Games and World Championships) in a recent study (Healy et al., 2019). The sprint times were measured either by high-speed videography or a laser device, or a combination of the two (Healy et al., 2019). The mean sprint times, in 10-m increments, and the mean sprint speeds (termed velocities in the study of Healy et al. (2019) but speeds here due to equivalence), in 20-m increments, up to 80 m are presented in Table 11.1. Also shown in Table 11.1, is the formula used to calculate the presented sprint speeds. Note how the sprint speeds were calculated between incrementally larger pairs of distances rather than always including the starting distance of zero (e.g., between 20 and 40 m rather than 0 and 40 m). The approach shown in Table 11.1 and by Healy et al. (2019) illustrates how average speed changes over more acute portions of the overall sprint distance, allowing for a more comprehensive sprint profile of the athletes, which is the benefit of being able to assess sprint performance over multiple sub-distances. For example, if only the mean time taken to sprint from 0 to 80 m is provided, only the average sprint speed across the whole of this distance can be calculated (e.g., 9.75 m/s). This approach would not provide any indication of how speed changed over the course of the sprint (i.e., acceleration) or what the approximate maximal sprint speed attained by the athlete was and within which of the measured sub-distances it was achieved. This information is likely to be of primary interest to strength and conditioning and skills coaches who train track athletes, particularly sprinters.

Task 2: Calculating Sprint Acceleration

Because most team-sport athletes will not reach maximal sprint speeds during match play, their maximal sprint speeds over shorter, more representative distances, are more likely to be assessed. In a recent study conducted with male youth rugby players,

Table 11.1 Sprint times, split distances, and speeds of male 100-m sprinters.

Distance (m)	Sprint Times (s)	Distance (m)	Sprint Speeds (m/s)	Speed Calculation
10	1.752			
20	2.817	0–20	9.39	$= (20 - 0) \div (2.817 - 1.752)$
30	3.710			
40	4.665	20–40	10.82	$= (40 - 20) \div (4.665 - 2.817)$
50	5.467			
60	6.441	40–60	11.26	$= (60 - 40)/(6.441 - 4.665)$
70	7.186			
80	8.203	60–80	11.35	$= (80 - 60)/(8.203 - 6.441)$

Table 11.2 Sprint time, speed, and acceleration of male youth rugby players.

Distance (m)	Sprint Time (s)	Sprint Speed (m/s)	Sprint Acceleration (m/s²)	Acceleration Calculation
10	1.69	5.92	3.50	$= (5.92 - 0.00) \div (1.69 - 0.00)$
20	2.98	7.75	1.42	$= (7.75 - 5.92) \div (2.98 - 1.69)$
30	4.19	8.26	0.42	$= (8.26 - 7.75) \div (4.19 - 2.98)$
40	5.41	8.20	−0.06	$= (8.20 - 8.26) \div (5.41 - 4.19)$
50	6.64	8.13	−0.05	$= (8.13 - 8.20) \div (6.64 - 5.41)$

for example, the 10-, 20-, 30-, 40- and 50-m sprint times, as measured by ETGs, were reported (Zabaloy et al., 2021). The mean sprint times for the under 18-year-old backs are presented in Table 11.2. From the sprint times, we have calculated the sprint speeds, per the example shown in Task 1, and the sprint acceleration. Sprint acceleration is calculated as a change in velocity (or speed, if running in one direction) divided by change time between any two increments that we chose, so in 10-m increments along the 50-m sprint, in this example. We can see in Table 11.2 that sprint speed increases up to 30 m but begins to decrease somewhere between the 30- and 40-m interval and continues to do so between the 40- and 50-m interval. This reduction in sprint speed is reflected by the corresponding negative acceleration values, which reflects that the athletes were decelerating over the last two sprint intervals. These data indicate that under 18-year-old male rugby backs may, on average, attain their maximal sprint speed somewhere around 30 m.

Task 3: Calculating Sprint Momentum

A factor to consider when either monitoring within-athlete changes in sprint speed in response to training or competition, or comparing sprint speeds between athletes, is body mass. In regard to the latter application, the 5-, 10-, 20-, 30-, and 40-m sprint times, as measured by ETGs, were reported for international female rugby league players, comprised of both the back and forward positional sub-groups (Jones et al., 2016). The mean sprint times for each positional sub-group are presented in Table 11.3. From the sprint times, we have calculated the sprint speeds, per the example shown in Task 1. Like in the study by Zabaloy et al. (2021), sprint speed increased up to 30 m but began to decrease somewhere between the 30- and 40-m interval, for each group. The backs outperformed the forwards for sprint speed at every measured sprint distance. However, the mean body mass of the backs and forwards was 66 and 80.7 kg, respectively (Jones et al., 2016), which is typically expected. Sprint momentum is calculated by multiplying body mass by sprint speed and is thought to be important for collision-sport athletes, such as rugby league players (Baker and Newton, 2008). We calculated sprint momentum from the sprint speed data and showed the calculation for each sprint distance and positional sub-group in Table 11.3. As can be seen, the sprint momentum is larger for the forwards at every measured sprint distance. Thus, focussing on sprint times or speeds alone can provide a narrow perspective on a collision-sport athlete's sprint performance. Of course, sprint speed is still important for forwards, but so is sprint momentum, thus reporting the two side-by-side will arguably better inform the strength and conditioning coach of each athlete's upcoming training needs.

Table 11.3 Sprint time, speed, and momentum of international female rugby league players comprised of backs (top half) and forwards (bottom half).

Distance (m)	Sprint Time (s)	Sprint Speed (m/s)	Sprint Momentum (kg·m/s)	Momentum Calculation
5	1.07	4.67	308	= 66 × 4.67
10	1.87	6.25	413	= 66 × 6.25
20	3.36	6.71	443	= 66 × 6.71
30	4.68	7.58	500	= 66 × 7.58
40	6.13	6.90	455	= 66 × 6.90
5	1.17	4.27	345	= 80.7 × 4.27
10	2.01	5.95	480	= 80.7 × 5.95
20	3.60	6.29	508	= 80.7 × 6.29
30	5.05	6.90	557	= 80.7 × 6.90
40	6.59	6.49	524	= 80.7 × 6.49

Summary

It is important for most athletes to be able to attain high sprint speeds over various, match-specific, distances to reach the highest level within their sport. The device used by the strength and conditioning coach to measure sprint speed will likely depend on budget and/or availability but irrespective of the device used, they should dedicate sufficient time to become familiar with how to better use it within its limits and develop robust standardization procedures. Understanding how sprint speed was attained for different athletes and/or how it changed or remained the same after a period of training or competition by also reporting sprint acceleration and sprint momentum will likely be beneficial to the identification of upcoming training priorities.

References

Altmann, S., Hoffmann, M., Kurz, G., Neumann, R., Woll, A. & Haertel, S. 2015. Different starting distances affect 5-m sprint times. *J Strength Cond Res*, 29, 2361–6.

Ashton, J. & Jones, P. A. 2019. The reliability of using a laser device to assess deceleration ability. *Sports (Basel)*, 7.

Baena-Raya, A., Soriano-Maldonado, A., Rodríguez-Pérez, M. A., García-De-Alcaraz, A., Ortega-Becerra, M., Jiménez-Reyes, P. & García-Ramos, A. 2021. The force-velocity profile as determinant of spike and serve ball speed in top-level male volleyball players. *PLOS One*, 16, e0249612.

Baker, D. G. & Newton, R. U. 2008. Comparison of lower body strength, power, acceleration, speed, agility, and sprint momentum to describe and compare playing rank among professional rugby league players. *J Strength Cond Res*, 22, 153–8.

Beckerman, H., Roebroeck, M. E., Lankhorst, G. J., Becher, J. G., Bezemer, P. D. & Verbeek, A. L. M. 2001. Smallest real difference, a link between reproducibility and responsiveness. *Qual Life Res*, 10, 571–8.

Bezodis, N. E., Salo, A. I. & Trewartha, G. 2012. Measurement error in estimates of sprint velocity from a laser displacement measurement device. *Int J Sports Med*, 33, 439–44.

Buchheit, M. & Brown, M. 2020. Pre-season fitness testing in elite soccer: Integrating the 30–15 intermittent fitness test into the weekly microcycle. *Sport Perform Sci Rep*, 111, 1–3.

Carr, C., McMahon, J. J. & Comfort, P. 2015. Relationships between jump and sprint performance in first-class county cricketers. *J Trainol*, 4, 1–5.

Carr, C., McMahon, J. J. & Comfort, P. 2017. Changes in strength, power and speed across a season in English county cricketers. *Int J Sports Physiol Perform*, 12, 50–5.

Cronin, J. B., Green, J. P., Levin, G. T., Brughelli, M. E. & Frost, D. M. 2007. Effect of starting stance on initial sprint performance. *J Strength Cond Res*, 21, 990–2.

Dos'Santos, T., Thomas, C., Jones, P. A. & Comfort, P. 2017. Mechanical determinants of faster change of direction speed performance in male athletes. *J Strength Cond Res*, 31, 3, 696–705.

Duthie, G. M., Pyne, D. B., Ross, A. A., Livingstone, S. G. & Hooper, S. L. 2006. The reliability of ten-meter sprint time using different starting techniques. *J Strength Cond Res*, 20, 251.

Earp, J. E. & Newton, R. U. 2012. Advances in electronic timing systems: Considerations for selecting an appropriate timing system. *J Strength Cond Res*, 26, 1245–8.

Filter, A., Olivares-Jabalera, J., Santalla, A., Morente-Sánchez, J., Robles-Rodríguez, J., Requena, B. & Loturco, I. 2020. Curve sprinting in soccer: Kinematic and neuromuscular analysis. *Int J Sports Med*, 41, 744–50.

Fílter, A., Olivares, J., Santalla, A., Nakamura, F. Y., Loturco, I. & Requena, B. 2020. New curve sprint test for soccer players: Reliability and relationship with linear sprint. *J Sports Sci*, 38, 1320–5.

Foden, M., Astley, S., Comfort, P., McMahon, J. J., Matthews, M. & Jones, P. A. 2015. Relationships between speed, change of direction and jump performance with cricket specific speed tests in male academy cricketers. *J Trainol*, 4, 37–42.

Frost, D. M. & Cronin, J. B. 2011. Stepping back to improve sprint performance: A kinetic analysis of the first step forwards. *J Strength Cond Res*, 25, 2721–8.

Frost, D. M., Cronin, J. B. & Levin, G. 2008. Stepping backward can improve sprint performance over short distances. *J Strength Cond Res*, 22, 918–22.

Ghigiarelli, J. J., Ferrara, K. J., Poblete, K. M., Valle, C. F., Gonzalez, A. M. & Sell, K. M. 2022. Level of agreement, reliability, and minimal detectable change of the Musclelab™ laser speed device on Force–Velocity–Power sprint profiles in division II. Collegiate Athletes. *Sports*, 10, 57.

Haugen, T. & Buchheit, M. 2016. Sprint running performance monitoring: Methodological and practical considerations. *Sports Med*, 46, 641–56.

Haugen, T. A., Tønnessen, E. & Seiler, S. K. 2012. The difference is in the start: Impact of timing and start procedure on sprint running performance. *J Strength Cond Res*, 26, 473–9.

Haugen, T. A., Tønnessen, E., Svendsen, I. S. & Seiler, S. 2014. Sprint time differences between single- and dual-beam timing systems. *J Strength Cond Res*, 28, 2376–9.

Healy, R., Kenny, I. C. & Harrison, A. J. 2019. Profiling elite male 100-m sprint performance: The role of maximum velocity and relative acceleration. *J Sport Health Sci*.

Johnson, T. M., Brown, L. E., Coburn, J. W., Judelson, D. A., Khamoui, A. V., Tran, T. T. & Uribe, B. P. 2010. Effect of four different starting stances on sprint time in collegiate volleyball players. *J Strength Cond Res*, 24, 2641–6.

Jones, B., Emmonds, S., Hind, K., Nicholson, G., Rutherford, Z. & Till, K. 2016. Physical qualities of international female Rugby league players by playing position. *J Strength Cond Res*, 30, 1333–40.

Kobal, R., Freitas, T. T., Fílter, A., Requena, B., Barroso, R., Rossetti, M., Jorge, R. M., Carvalho, L., Pereira, L. A. & Loturco, I. 2021. Curve sprint in elite female soccer players: Relationship with linear sprint and jump performance. *Int J Environ Res Public Health*, 18, 2306.

Mann, J. B., Ivey, P. J., Brechue, W. F. & Mayhew, J. L. 2015. Validity and reliability of hand and electronic timing for 40-yd sprint in college football players. *J Strength Cond Res*, 29, 1509–14.

Munshi, P., Khan, M. H., Arora, N. K., Nuhmani, S., Anwer, S., Li, H. & Alghadir, A. H. 2022. Effects of plyometric and whole-body vibration on physical performance in collegiate basketball players: A crossover randomized trial. *Sci Rep*, 12, 1–9.

Ripley, N., Comfort, P. & McMahon, J. J. 2020. Retention of adaptations to eccentric hamstring strength and bicep femoris fascicle length from a 7-week sprint or Nordic training intervention. *J Strength Cond Res*, 35, e221–2.

Romero-Franco, N., Jiménez-Reyes, P., Castaño-Zambudio, A., Capelo-Ramírez, F., Rodríguez-Juan, J. J., González-Hernández, J., Toscano-Bendala, F. J., Cuadrado-Peñafiel, V. & Balsalobre-Fernández, C. 2017. Sprint performance and mechanical outputs computed with an iPhone app: Comparison with existing reference methods. *Eur J Sport Sci*, 17, 386–92.

Salo, A. & Bezodis, I. 2004. Which starting style is faster in sprint running standing or crouch start? *Sports Biomech*, 3, 43–54.

Yeadon, M. R., Kato, T. & Kerwin, D. G. 1999. Measuring running speed using photocells. *J Sports Sci*, 17, 249–57.

Zabaloy, S., Giráldez, J., Gazzo, F., Villaseca-Vicuña, R. & González, J. G. 2021. In-season assessment of sprint speed and sprint momentum in Rugby players according to the age category and playing position. *J Hum Kinet*, 77, 274–86.

Zaragoza, J. A., Johson, Q. R., Lawson, D. J., Alfaro, E. L., Dawes, J. J. & Smith, D. B. 2022. Relationships between lower-body power, sprint and change of direction speed among collegiate basketball players by sex. *Int J Exerc Sci*, 15, 974–84.

12 Change of Direction Performance

Paul Comfort and John McMahon

Part 1: Introduction

The ability to change direction efficiently and effectively is extremely important in many team and court-based sports, due to the frequent alterations in movement patterns, including decelerations and changes of direction (Brughelli et al., 2008; Barber et al., 2016; Taylor et al., 2017). For example, in soccer, players reportedly change direction every 4–6 seconds (Stolen et al., 2005), with an average of 727 ± 203 changes of direction per match, in the English Premier League (Bloomfield et al., 2007). While many of the changes of direction may not be too demanding (e.g., ~600 <90°), more demanding changes of direction (e.g., 90–180°) are performed by each athlete ~90 times per match (Bloomfield et al., 2007). Similarly, professional netball players have been reported to change direction or activity pattern on average every 6 seconds (Davidson and Trewartha, 2008; Chandler et al., 2014).

Change of direction (CoD) and agility should not be confused or used interchangeably, as agility has been defined as "a rapid and accurate whole-body movement, with change of velocity or direction, in response to a stimulus" (Sheppard and Young, 2006), with CoD being pre-planned and therefore not in response to a stimulus. As such, the majority of tests which include *"agility"* in the title are simply tests of CoD performance, with performance evaluated based on time to completion. While an agility test may seem more specific to sporting scenarios and include a cognitive component, there are limitations with such assessments, with the primary limitation being that the stimuli used are not the movement of an opponent (how would this be standardized for a test?), but commonly a flashing light, sound (e.g., whistle, or coach shouting a direction), or an arrow on a screen. In addition, if an athlete demonstrates poor performance during an agility task, it is difficult to determine if this was due to a delay in the decision-making process (i.e., cognitive), or the physical capability to perform the task, without assessing CoD performance in a similar task.

Nimphius et al. (2018) explain that a CoD test should assess the individual's ability to decelerate and reaccelerate for a specific direction change, without evaluating the other physical qualities, e.g., maximal velocity or endurance. As such, some commonly used CoD tests have notable limitations commonly based around test duration and the associated metabolic demands (Table 12.1). For a detailed evaluation of assessments, CoD, and agility assessments, see Jones and Nimphius (2019).

When selecting the appropriate CoD test, it is important to consider the demands of the sport and the CoD actions performed. For example, the 505 CoD tests include a 180° turn, which can commonly be seen in sports such as cricket (e.g., changing

DOI: 10.4324/9781003186762-12

Table 12.1 Comparison of a selection of common change of direction tests.

Test	CoD angle	Distance	time to Completion	Response to stimulus
Modified 505	180°	10 m	2.5–3.0 s	✗
Traditional 505	180°	10 m*	~3.0 s	✗
L Run	180°	~27 m	7.0–8.0 s	✗
Illinois Agility Test	180°	~60 m	13–19 s	✗
T-test	90°	36.56 m	7.5–13 s	✗
Pro-Agility Test	180°	~18 m	4.0–5.0 s	✗
Y-Agility Test	~45°	8–11 m	1.5–2.5 s	✓

Modified from Jones and Nimphius (2019).

*Timed distance (does not include initial 10 m approach).

direction between wickets) and rugby league (e.g., when the defending retreat 10 metres from the tackle prior to the next play of the ball) and is clearly an important physical quality to evaluate, with the demand of the turn being similar to those in the sport. However, with longer duration tests, such as the "Illinois *Agility* Test," it can be difficult to determine whether the athlete is limited by their ability to perform at high intensities for the duration of the test, or whether their performance is limited due to poor acceleration, poor deceleration or their technique (Nimphius et al., 2018; Jones and Nimphius, 2019).

Part 2: Change of Direction Assessments

Change of direction tests such as the 505 and modified 505 are effective at evaluating an athlete's ability to accelerate, decelerate, change direction, and reaccelerate, which is important in all multidirectional sports (Nimphius et al., 2018; Dos'santos et al., 2020; Ryan et al., 2022c). However, calculation of the change of direction deficit (CoDD) (time to complete the 505 test – maximal 10-m sprint time) may be more insightful than simply considering the time to complete the CoD test, as the deficit score indicates the additional time required to decelerate, turn (change direction) and re-accelerate. Because the modified 505 CoD test includes two 5-m accelerations (Figure 12.1), it may be more appropriate to calculate the CoDD by doubling the 5-m sprint time and subtracting that value from the time to complete the CoD test, resulting in a deficit which represents the individual's time to decelerate at the end of the initial 5 m and turn; however, no research regarding this appears to have been published. Cuthbert et al. (2019) have also demonstrated that the CoDD calculation can reliably be applied to a CoD test involving a 90° cut.

Ryan et al. (2022a, 2022b) have also suggested subdividing the phases of the modified 505 CoD test further to consider performance of the acceleration, deceleration, 180° turn, and the reacceleration phases. This can be achieved by adding two additional sets of timing gates to provide five split times (Figure 12.2). It should be noted, however, that there is currently limited published normative data to make comparisons to. Additionally, it is possible that the third set of timing gates (immediately pre-/post-CoD) may be too close to the CoD line for the athlete to clear the laser beam when they change direction (i.e., perform the 180° turn) and then retrigger it as the commence reacceleration.

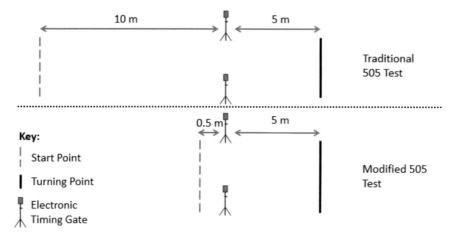

Figure 12.1 Comparison of the traditional and modified 505 change of direction tests.

5-0-5 Change of Direction

As with the assessment of sprint speed (Chapter 11), electronic timing gates (ETG) should be used to evaluate CoD performance based on the time to complete the test. For the traditional 505 CoD test, the ETG should be set up 10 m from the start line and 5 m from the turn line (Figure 12.2), at a height which approximately resembles hip height for the athlete(s). The athlete should start in a 2-point stance with their front foot on the start line and be instructed to accelerate maximally through the initial 10+ metres and then decelerate and change direction with their desired foot contacting the turn line, when making the 180° turn, followed by another maximal acceleration back through the ETG. If the athlete does not appear to accelerate maximally across the initial 10 m (i.e., adopting a pacing strategy), or starts to decelerate prior to passing through the 5-m ETG after the turn, the trial should be discounted and repeated.

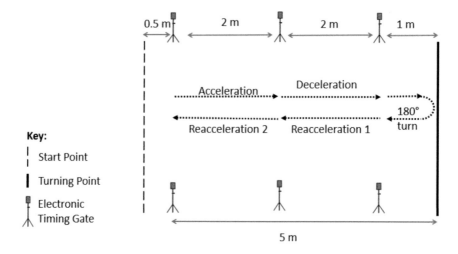

Figure 12.2 Subdivision of the modified 505 change of direction test to provide additional phase-specific information as suggested by Ryan et al. (2022a, 2022b).

Ideally, when assessing groups of athletes, they can rotate between trials to ensure a minimum of a 60 s rest between efforts, in an attempt to mitigate fatigue. The athletes should complete three acceptable trials per leg (e.g., three trials changing direction with the final foot contact on the turn line for both left and right legs), with the mean of the three trials taken forward for analysis.

To calculate the 505 CoD deficit, take the 505 duration and subtract the 10-m sprint time. Please note that in an ideal testing battery, the sports scientist/strength and conditioning coach would evaluate linear sprint performance prior to the traditional 505 CoD test so that they know the athletes' 10-m sprint time and can easily determine if they are adopting a pacing strategy.

Data Interpretation

It is important to consider how an athlete's performance compares to published normative performances, although one should be mindful that there may be subtle differences in the testing procedures (e.g., distances measured in yards or metres, positioning of ETG) which may affect the comparisons. In addition, the data should be considered in relation to the changes in the athlete's performance in other tasks, such as 5-m and 10-m sprint performances, as a higher speed during short sprints will result in a greater momentum, making the deceleration and CoD (i.e., turn) more challenging. Alternatively, if the athlete's mass has increased over time, their momentum will also increase, even if their sprint speeds have not increased. Collect some data and compare their performances to the normative data below, or any normative data that you can find in the published research (Table 12.2). Then try and determine if the athlete should focus on increasing linear sprint speed, or CoD performance, based on the overall CoD time and the CoDD. It will also be worth considering the 5-m and 10-m sprint times in conjunction with this data.

Modified 5-0-5 Change of Direction

For the modified 505 CoD test, the ETG should be set up 0.5 m from the start line and 5 m from the turn line (Figure 12.2), at a height which approximately resembles hip height for the athlete(s). The athlete should start in a 2-point stance with their front foot on the start line and be instructed to accelerate maximally through the

Table 12.2 Example normative data for the traditional 505 and 505 deficit for a range of sports.

Sport	CoD Time (s)	CoDD (s)	Compare Your Data	
			CoD Time (s)	CoDD (s)
Soccer	2.34 ± 0.12 s	/		
Basketball	2.43 ± 0.18 s	/		
Rugby League	2.34 ± 0.20 s	/		
Lacrosse	2.50 ± 0.20 s	/		
Rugby Union	2.48 ± 0.11 s	/		
Tennis	2.50 ± 0.13 s	0.52 ± 0.10 s		
Netball	2.40 ± 0.12 s	0.62 ± 0.07 s		
Cricket	2.50 ± 0.10 s	0.62 ± 0.07 s		

CoD = Change of direction; CoDD = Change of direction deficit.

initial 10+ metres and then decelerate and change direction with their desired foot contacting the turn line, when making the 180° turn, followed by another maximal acceleration back through the ETG. If the athlete starts to decelerate prior to passing through the 5 m ETG after the turn, the trial should be discounted and repeated.

Ideally, when assessing groups of athletes, they can rotate between trials to ensure a minimum of a 60 s rest between efforts, in an attempt to mitigate fatigue. The athletes should complete three acceptable trials per leg (e.g., three trials changing direction with the final foot contact on the turn line for both left and right legs), with the mean of the three trials taken forward for analysis. To calculate the modified 505 CoDD, take the modified 505 duration and subtract the 10-m sprint time.

Data Interpretation

As mentioned previously, it is important to consider how an athlete's performances compare to published normative performances, although you should be mindful that there may be subtle differences in the testing procedures (e.g., distance that the athlete starts from the timing gates which can vary between 0.3 m, 0.5 m, and 1 m) which may affect the comparisons due to differences in approach speed. In addition, the data should be considered in relation to the changes in the athlete's performance in other tasks, such as 5-m sprint performance, as a higher speed results in a greater momentum, making the deceleration and CoD (i.e., turn) more challenging. Alternatively, if the athlete's mass has increased over time, their momentum will also increase, even if their sprint speeds have not increased. Collect some data and compare their performances to the normative data below, or any normative data that you can find in the published research (Table 12.3). Then try and determine if the athlete should focus on increasing linear sprint speed, or CoD performance, based on the overall CoD time and the CoDD. It will also be worth considering your 5-m sprint times in conjunction with this data.

T-Test

The t-test (also incorrectly referred to as the *agility* t-test) is commonly used to assess CoD performance across numerous sports, although it is somewhat under-researched. It is sometimes more appropriately referred to as a test of manoeuvrability and is seen by some as more specific to common movement patterns observed in team sports as it includes forward running, side shuffling, and backpedalling to complete the T-shaped course. When selecting the appropriate CoD test, practitioners should consider if the test reflects some of the common movement patterns in the sport, with

Table 12.3 Example normative data for the modified 505 test for a range of sports.

| Sport | CoD time (s) | CoDD (s) | Compare your data | |
			CoD time (s)	CoDD (s)
Rugby League	2.66 ± 0.14 s	/		
Tennis	2.68 ± 0.13 s	/		
Cricket	2.70 ± 0.15 s	/		

CoD = Change of direction; CoDD = Change of direction deficit.

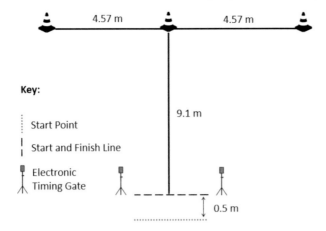

Figure 12.3 T-test set-up.

the t-test clearly appropriate for sports such as volleyball (Gabbett and Georgieff, 2007; Melrose et al., 2007) and numerous racket sports.

The test has been shown to be highly reliable (intraclass correlation coefficient = 0.82–0.96) with the smallest detectable difference of ~3.7% and ~5.4% in females and males, respectively (Munro and Herrington, 2011). As such, when assessing individual athletes, changes greater than these magnitudes can be considered a real change, although Munro and Herrington (2011) suggested that four trials should be performed and the initial trial should be disregarded, as there is a learning effect which stabilizes after the first trial.

The t-test should be set up as originally described by Semenick (1990), although timing should be conducted using ETG rather than a stopwatch (Figure 12.3). The course, as the name suggests, resembles a T, with the timing gates at the start/finish point and the initial cone 9.14 m from the start line, with two further cones 4.57 m to the left and right of the first cone. Athletes should start in a 2-point stance 0.5 m behind the ETG to prevent a false trigger of the timing system, although some researchers have used 0.3 m (Pereira et al., 2018), this can occasionally result in a false trigger, especially in larger athletes. The athlete should sprint to the first cone, touching it with the tip of their right hand and then shuffle to the left to touch the cone with their left hand, shuffle to the right 9.14 m to touch the cone with their right hand, shuffle 4.57 m back to the middle cone with their left hand and then backpedal until they pass through the timing gates (Pauole et al., 2000; Munro and Herrington, 2011). As already mentioned, four trials should be performed with the initial trial discounted and a mean of the final three trials used for analysis, as the initial trial has been shown to result in a learning effect (Munro and Herrington, 2011).

L-Run

The L-run is also referred to as the 3-cone drill (Sierer et al., 2008; Robbins, 2010; Nimphius et al., 2016) and has been used extensively in the American Football as part of the combine (Sierer et al., 2008; Robbins, 2010; Fitzgerald and Jensen, 2020). Researchers have reported good reliability (intraclass correlation coefficients of 0.80

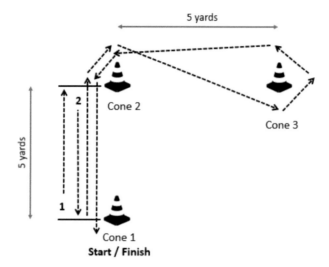

Figure 12.4 L-Run (a.k.a. 3 cone drill) sequence. The athlete performing a shuttle run between cones 1 and 2, touching the cone 2 line with their left hand prior to returning to cone 1, then sprints back to and around cone 2 in a clockwise fashion, with the cone on their right side, then counter-clock-wise around cone 3 with the cone on their left side, back around cone 2 with the cone on their left and finally back across the line at cone 1 to finish. Performance is evaluated based on time to completion.

and 0.88 for males and females, respectively), and low variability (coefficient of variation 1.63–2.23%) (Stewart et al., 2014). Interestingly, the movements involved do not appear to follow the sequence of movements observed in numerous sports. Similar to the t-test, this can be considered a test of manoeuvrability due to the movement patterns involved, where the athlete performs a shuttle run between cones 1 and 2, touching the cone 2 line with their left hand prior to returning to cone 1, then sprints back to and around cone 2 in a clockwise fashion, with the cone on their right side, then counter-clock-wise around cone 3 with the cone on their left side, back around cone 2 with the cone on their left and finally back across the line at cone 1 to finish (Figure 12.4). Performance is evaluated based on time to completion, with timing ideally determined using ETG set at the start/finish line.

Case Study

Below is a case study of a rugby union full-back through pre-season (6 weeks) and the start of the competitive season (4 weeks). Baseline performance at the start of pre-season was considered adequate (Table 12.4), with the primary training focus on enhancing maximal and rapid force production, to improve acceleration (short sprint performance) and CoD performance.

The focus of the gym-based training during the first 6 weeks of pre-season was to maximize force production (using high loads [≥85% one repetition maximum] and moderate volumes [3–5 sets of 3–5 repetitions per exercise] and ensure good movement quality during the lower limb control-focused exercises and the ballistic and plyometric (reactive) tasks. During the 4 weeks at the start of the season, sessions

Table 12.4 Changes in physical characteristics of a rugby union player over two phases of training.

		Start of Pre-season (W0)	End of Pre-season (W6)	In Season (W10)
Body Mass (kg)		94.5	94.0	94.0
Body Fat (%)		10.2	8.1	8.3
Sprint	5 m (s)	1.09	0.95	0.96
	10 m (s)	1.78	1.69	1.65
	20 m (s)	3.12	2.98	2.89
5-0-5 CoD (s)		2.78	2.75	2.62
5-0-5 CoDD (s)		1.00	1.06	0.97
1RM Back Squat (kg/kg)		1.71	1.95	/
IMTP	PF (N/kg)	39.1	47.0	47.2
	F150 (N/kg)	24.8	27.3	29.0
	F250 (N/kg)	32.9	35.6	36.5

CoD = Change of direction (modified 5-0-5); CoDD = Change of direction deficit (5-0-5 time – 10-m sprint time); RM = Repetition maximum; IMTP = Isometric mid-thigh pull; PF = Peak force; F150 = force at 150 ms; F250 = Force at 250 ms.

alternated between a strength-speed and speed strength emphasis. Notable improvements in 5-m and 10-m sprint performances can be seen across the pre-season period, but minimal change in 505 CoD performance and an increase in the CoDD, which is likely due to the increased momentum due to an increased sprint speed. In contrast, by week 10 (after the first 4 weeks of the season), 5-m and 10-m sprint performance has not changed notably, but the athlete now demonstrates improvements in 505 CoD performance and likely due to a decrease in the CoDD due to an improved ability to decelerate and turn (i.e., change direction). This is commonly observed in numerous collision sports and practitioners should be aware of the potential initial decrease in CoD performance when short sprint performance initially increases.

References

Barber, O. R., Thomas, C., Jones, P. A., Mcmahon, J. J. & Comfort, P. 2016. Reliability of the 505 change-of-direction test in netball players. *Int J Sports Physiol Perform*, 11, 377–80.

Bloomfield, J., Polman, R. & O'donoghue, P. 2007. Physical demands of different positions in FA premier league soccer. *J Sports Sci Med*, 6, 63–70.

Brughelli, M., Cronin, J., Levin, G. & Chaouachi, A. 2008. Understanding change of direction ability in sport. *Sports Med*, 38, 1045–63.

Chandler, P. T., Pinder, S. J., Curran, J. D. & Gabbett, T. J. 2014. Physical demands of training and competition in collegiate netball players. *J Strength Cond Res*, 28, 2732–7.

Cuthbert, M., Thomas, C., Dos'santos, T. & Jones, P. A. 2019. Application of change of direction deficit to evaluate cutting ability. *J Strength Cond Res*, 33, 2138–44.

Davidson, A. & Trewartha, G. 2008. Understanding the physiological demands of netball: A time-motion investigation. *Int J Perform Anal Sport*, 8, 1–17.

Dos'santos, T., McBurnie, A., Thomas, C., Comfort, P. & Jones, P. A. 2020. Biomechanical determinants of the modified and traditional 505 change of direction speed test. *J Strength Cond Res*, 34, 1285–96.

Fitzgerald, C. F. & Jensen, R. L. 2020. A comparison of the national football league's annual national football league combine 1999–2000 to 2015–2016. *J Strength Cond Res*, 34, 771–8.

Gabbett, T. & Georgieff, B. 2007. Physiological and anthropometric characteristics of Australian junior national, state, and novice volleyball players. *J Strength Cond Res*, 21, 902–8.

Jones, P. A. & Nimphius, S. 2019. Change of direction and agility. In: Comfort, P., Jones, P. A. & McMahon, J. J. (eds) *Performance Assessment in Strength and Conditioning*. Abingdon, UK: Routledge.

Melrose, D. R., Spaniol, F. J., Bohling, M. E. & Bonnette, R. A. 2007. Physiological and performance characteristics of adolescent club volleyball players. *J Strength Cond Res*, 21, 481–6.

Munro, A. G. & Herrington, L. C. 2011. Between-session reliability of four hop tests and the agility t-test. *J Strength Cond Res*, 25, 1470–7.

Nimphius, S., Callaghan, S. J., Bezodis, N. E. & Lockie, R. G. 2018. Change of direction and agility tests: Challenging our current measures of performance. *Strength Cond J*, 40, 26–38.

Nimphius, S., Callaghan, S. J., Spiteri, T. & Lockie, R. G. 2016. Change of direction deficit: A more isolated measure of change of direction performance than total 505 times. *J Strength Cond Res*, 30, 3024–32.

Pauole, K., Madole, K., Garhammer, J., Lacourse, M. & Rozenek, R. 2000. Reliability and validity of the t-test as a measure of agility, leg power, and leg speed in college-aged men and women. *J Strength Cond Res*, 14, 443–50.

Pereira, L. A., Nimphius, S., Kobal, R., Kitamura, K., Turisco, L. A. L., Orsi, R. C., Cal Abad, C. C. & Loturco, I. 2018. Relationship between change of direction, speed, and power in male and female national Olympic team handball athletes. *J Strength Cond Res*, 32, 2987–94.

Robbins, D. W. 2010. The national football league (NFL) combine: Does normalized data better predict performance in the NFL draft? *J Strength Cond Res*, 24, 2888–99.

Ryan, C., Uthoff, A., Mckenzie, C. & Cronin, J. 2022a. New perspectives of the traditional and modified 5-0-5 change of direction test. *Strength Cond J*, E-pub ahead of print.

Ryan, C., Uthoff, A., Mckenzie, C. & Cronin, J. 2022b. Sub-phase analysis of the modified 5-0-5 test for better change of direction diagnostics. *J Sport Exer Sci*, 6, 16–21.

Ryan, C., Uthoff, A., Mckenzie, C. & Cronin, J. 2022c. Traditional and modified 5-0-5 change of direction test: Normative and reliability analysis. *Strength Cond J*, 44, 22–37.

Semenick, D. 1990. Tests and measurements: The t-test. *Strength Cond J*, 12, 36–7.

Sheppard, J. & Young, W. 2006. Agility literature review: Classifications, training and testing. *J Sports Sci*, 24, 919–32.

Sierer, S. P., Battaglini, C. L., Mihalik, J. P., Shields, E. W. & Tomasini, N. T. 2008. The national football league combine: Performance differences between drafted and nondrafted players entering the 2004 and 2005 drafts. *J Strength Cond Res*, 22, 6–12.

Stewart, P. F., Turner, A. N. & Miller, S. C. 2014. Reliability, factorial validity, and interrelationships of five commonly used change of direction speed tests. *Scand J Med Sci Sports*, 24, 500–6.

Stolen, T., Chamari, K., Castagna, C. & Wisloff, U. 2005. Physiology of soccer: An update. *Sports Med*, 35, 501–36.

Taylor, J. B., Wright, A. A., Dischiavi, S. L., Townsend, M. A. & Marmon, A. R. 2017. Activity demands during multi-directional team sports: A systematic review. *Sports Med*, 47, 2533–51.

Index

Note: Page references in *italics* denote figures and in **bold** denote tables.

For Product Safety Concerns and Information please contact our
EU representative GPSR@taylorandfrancis.com Taylor & Francis
Verlag GmbH, Kaufingerstraße 24, 80331 München, Germany